THE
BUSINESSMAN'S
DIET

THE BUSINESSMAN'S DIET

Michael Teff

PIATKUS

First published in
Great Britain in 1988 by
Judy Piatkus (Publishers) Ltd,
5 Windmill Street, London W1P 1HF

British Library Cataloguing in Publication Data

Teff, Michael, *1932 –*
  The businessman's diet.
  1. Physical fitness. Slimming. Diet
  I. Title
  613.2′5

  ISBN 0–86188–700–X

Edited by Susan Fleming
Illustrations by Mike Dickinson
Design by Sue Ryall

Phototypeset by Action Typesetting Limited, Gloucester
Printed and bound in Great Britain by
Billing & Sons Ltd, Worcester

CONTENTS

Acknowledgements

A heart-felt thank-you to all those friends and clients (not always synonymous) whose experiences and anecdotes I shamelessly exposed.

Special gratitude to Dr. Sally Birkett, Margaret Birkett, Moira Johnston, Jenny Cowgill, Susan Fleming, Karen Game, Eden Phillips, Karen Mottram, Caroline Cumberbatch, Lady Jean Rowe, Ros Schwartz, Dr. P. H. Wise, and Gill Cormode at Piatkus.

Introduction

You're a businessman. Every day you make practical decisions. You consider the pros and cons of varied propositions, you plan financial investments, look to the long term, and base those decisions on the potential profit and loss.

Initial investment in The Businessman's Diet is miniscule – and in fact the decrease in your life-insurance premiums could be ten times the cost of the book itself. The investment in terms of planning, charting and consulting is moderate.

Potential losses occur both in the short and long term. You'll lose that bulge around the tummy and that second chin that's just starting to appear. You'll certainly lose weight in general – and *keep* it off.

The potential profits are enormous – a slimmer, healthier body, a longer and happier life to enjoy your family, and a marvellous sense of well-being. In short, you'll be fulfilling your potential – to yourself, and to all those around you.

One of your greatest assets is your partner, and indeed it may be your partner who is investigating the potential of this investment for you. Although most of the work involved is to be done by you, it's your partner upon whom your ultimate success depends.

The Businessman's Diet *does* work. It's sensible and successful, and one which takes full account of every aspect of your business life. You start off with a basic programme for a fortnight which will cut out certain foods, but will not cut down on food *quantity*. You'll never feel hungry. Thereafter, there's a fortnight's bonus programme which allows you several perks or rewards. In tandem with some gentle or more robust exercises — depending on your initial fitness — your weight and shape should naturally and healthily change.

However, the programme can't work by itself. It needs you and your partner at every stage — to plan, to consult, to achieve. Perhaps the 'bottom line' is an unfortunate phrase to use in the context of a diet book, and I certainly can't guarantee a Paul Newman at the end of it all. But with the three of us — myself, you and your partner — working together, the result will be a slimmer, healthier and — dare I say it — sexier businessman.

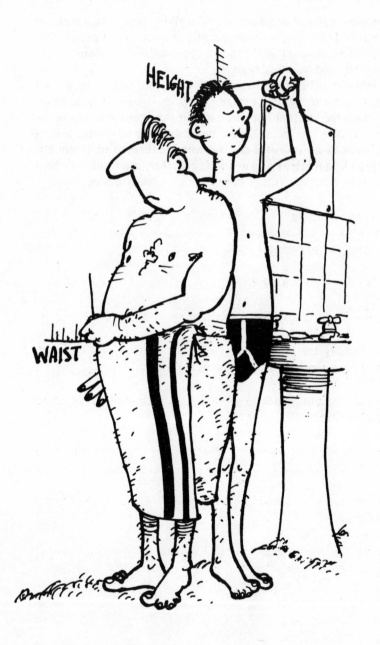

CHAPTER 1

The Moment of Truth

It's early morning. You've been to the loo and had your shower. Just the time to take a look at yourself in a full-length mirror — in the nude, of course.

Is this where you are NOW?

★ Having difficulty doing up the zip of your trousers?

★ Blaming the shirt-makers when the buttons pop off quite regularly (especially around the waist)?

★ Finding excuses not to go swimming with the family — 'too cold' perhaps?

★ Utilising three wardrobes of suits — large, larger and what you're wearing now?

★ Undoing your trousers — just a little — before getting into the driver's seat?

★ Raiding the fridge at midnight for that left-over slice of cake or perfect bit of Brie?

★ Regularly reaching for those anti-acid tablets on your bedside table?

If that's where you are NOW this is where you could be in four weeks or four months or four years:

★ Leading a fully active business and social life, physically and mentally.

★ Being there to enjoy your family – your wife and children *and* your grand-children and great-grand-children.

★ Looking and feeling healthy – energetic, attractive and confident.

★ Being easier to live with, be with and share with.

★ Maximising your business acumen – making quicker decisions and more decisive ones.

★ Taking full advantage of all life's pleasures – food and drink, travel, sport, the arts . . . and sex.

MOTIVATION

The first thing you need in order to to diet successfully is motivation, and motivation is very personal. Whatever your doctor may advise or your family urge, the decision to diet must come from you. Failing a medical examination for life insurance, or catching sight of yourself in the bathroom mirror, may give the necessary impetus. Fear and vanity are powerful masters!

To press home the 'health' aspect, I've compiled a list of some of the illnesses and other horrors that can be caused by obesity. Disaster may not strike tomorrow, but it is much more likely to strike sometime in the future if you don't look after yourself *now*.

High blood pressure and diabetes, both of which can lead to heart attacks and angina.

Backache, varicose veins, pain or arthritis in ankles or knees.

Constipation, piles and diverticulitis, digestive and metabolic disorders.

Gallstones, cancer of the gall bladder, strokes and thrombosis.

Tooth decay, shortness of breath, sexual problems and lack of confidence.

Unpleasant reading, but true.

LET'S DISPOSE OF THE ALTERNATIVES FIRST

The quackery that goes on in the diet world is appalling, with enormous claims made for the value of certain crash diets, injections, pills, and supplements.

Whether you swallow different multi-coloured pills until you rattle, try to live on nothing but fruit, or water, or apples, or cheese, or whisky, or grapefruit, or eggs for ten days, supplement your meals with products with the appetising appeal of mattress stuffing, get yourself hypnotised and analysed, have your jaws wired, your stomach stapled, have a stomach by-pass operation, IN THE LONG RUN IT JUST WON'T WORK.

Yet no matter how bizarre the format, and no matter how much medical and dietary opinion opposes them, 'miracle cures' appear to have a ready market.

The fact is that any diet or programme that doesn't educate you to eat and drink so that you can control your weight successfully in the real world isn't worth a damn. And when I say the real world, I mean a normal, everyday existence with normal, everyday foods available to normal, everyday shoppers.

Pill-popping, injections, chemicals, what are you doing to yourself? And when the two-week course is up, or the supplements run out, you'll return to square one, and you're no wiser. So it's back to your previous eating pattern, and the weight comes on again – often more than when you began.

So what about these special low calorie diets, do I hear you ask? There's a great deal of controversy raging about the value of the so-called very low calorie diets available in health food stores and through networks of 'counsellors'. The American authorities have actually banned extremely low calorie diets and have insisted that their calorific value be increased dramatically; in one instance, more than doubled. In Britain and Europe there is considerable concern over their use and promotion, and warnings on advertisements may be strengthened.

Doctors, dieticians and health professionals have argued for years that the only way to lose weight is to educate yourself on what to eat, when to eat, and how much to eat. That's what you're going to do now.

SO, WHAT IS THIS BOOK SELLING?

On The Businessman's Diet, there are no gurus or miracles, there is no moralising, boredom or starvation. What you *do* get is:

★ A simple eating plan that you can live *and* work with, containing plenty of good, natural and easily available food that you can eat when you want to. Sure, you'll have an appetite for those foods and drinks you're missing – and *you'll* know what they are – but that's strictly an *appetite*, not a *hunger*.

★ A programme on which you'll never feel *hungry*. In fact, you might be eating far more than you have in the past and *you'll still lose weight*.

★ A diet based on weighing foods, not counting calories. The first part of the programme is based on approximately 1,000 calories a day; the bonus programme on 1,500. I realise that the initial weighing of foods is tiresome but you soon learn to judge it fairly accurately and it's certainly preferable to a continual calculation of calories. If I did advise sticking to, say, 1,000 calories per day, how am I to know you wouldn't rush out and blow the whole 1,000 calories on a couple of chocolate bars?

★ Lots of encouragement and plenty of tips.

★ A saving on £s as well as pounds. For instance, a man of 54 who is more than 28lb (12.5kg) over acceptable medical standards pays 30 per cent more in insurance premiums. You'll save the price of this book many times over.

It's not easy to change your lifestyle regarding food and drink, but it can be done if you approach it in a pragmatic, realistic and, dare I say, sober manner. What I'm suggesting is that you approach your eating habits in much the same way as you approach any business campaign. Think about it.

★ What is the ultimate or long-term objective?

★ What is the past history?

★ What is the current position?

★ Where do the benefits lie?

★ Where do the problems occur?

★ When do the problems occur?

★ Who should be involved in solutions?

★ What is a realistic target?

★ How long should a solution take?

Charting your progress and pin-pointing the problems are dealt with in Chapter 3. A table of acceptable weights according to your height appears on page 19, followed by charts on which you can fill in your individual measurements charting your changing shape as you follow the diet throughout the first four weeks. Whether your weight well exceeds the acceptable, or if you plan to lose only a few pounds, The Businessman's Diet is for you.

Even though the programme is based solely on simple and healthy everyday foods, it's always wise to check with your medical adviser beforehand. If you're diabetic, for instance – as I am – The Businessman's Diet is perfectly suitable for you with *no* exceptions. Two informative booklets for insulin-dependent and non-insulin-dependent diabetics will be most helpful. They're entitled 'Knowing about Diabetes', and are by Dr P. H. Wise, of the Diabetic and Endocrine Clinic, Charing Cross Hospital (published by W. Foulsham & Co. Ltd).

INITIAL PLANNING

Preparing yourself for the off is important, and it's not just a question of 'What the hell, I might as well have a go, what have I got to lose?'

What you're going to lose primarily is weight, so set yourself a realistic target. The weight chart on page 19 is the one I always use and it gives you a good indication of what your weight should be according to your height (I'm assuming that you're over 21 years old). If the chart indicates that you should weigh between 154 lb or 11 stone (69.9 kg) and 184 lb or 13 stone 2 lb (83.5 kg), and you're *over* that, your initial target weight should be the maximum – ie 13 stone 2 lb (83.5 kg). If, however, you presently weigh the maximum for that height, don't aim *below* the minimum; head for the middle of your weight band.

Never reach for the impossible or, more importantly, the un-maintainable. (The fact that you're big-boned, small-wristed or descend from a long line of men with large tummies makes a minimal difference and has been taken into account in the suggested weight targets.)

What you're also going to lose is a good few hours while planning and revising your food habits and – to a lesser extent – your lifestyle. For a start, for the week or so before you take the plunge, it's a good idea to keep a record of what you eat and drink *normally*. Fill this in on the chart on pages 22-23, and you'll then be able to see when your danger eating times are, what your danger foods are, and just how hard you might have to work to change on the basic weight-control programme. I do this with my personal clients, and it's very revelatory *if* they're honest with me and themselves! Don't ever go along with the self-delusion that if no-one sees you eat, it didn't happen. Be brutally honest.

While you are assessing your food intake, make a note of how and why you eat. It will be interesting – and informative – reading.

★ Do you only eat when you are hungry?

★ Do you eat when you are alone?

★ Do you eat when you are bored/nervous/angry/depressed?

★ Do you eat when you are watching television?

★ Do you eat when you are in the car?

★ Do you always sit down to eat?

★ Do you always finish everything on your plate? And everyone else's plates?

★ Do you ever refuse a second helping?

★ Do you always have something to eat mid-morning and mid-afternoon to get you through the day?

★ Do you raid the fridge the moment you get home?

★ Do you eat quickly so no-one will notice how much you eat?

★ Do you nibble when you drink?

Plan your new food programme as you would any other commercial project. Consult your partner at every stage, and that includes business partners – your secretary or PA who is such an integral part of your office life. It's your PA who keeps a continual eye on you during the day, and it's she or he who can be invaluable to your success.

If you're getting the back-up at home as well as the office, you're half-way there. Keep everyone who can help completely in the picture: don't just assume they know what you are planning. Children, for instance, are amazingly effective watchdogs when they know what Dad's allowed to eat, and particularly what *not* to eat. They'll guard the fridge with the tenacity of the SAS, and keep an eagle eye on your plate at mealtimes.

You need the support of the entire team:

★ Your loving partner at home

★ Your children

★ Your business assistant/s

★ Your firm's catering person

★ The proprietors of your favourite restaurants — whether for domestic dining-out or for business meals.

Don't be embarrassed to ask for help either, you're not losing one tiny bit of your masculinity or self-confidence. You're showing that you're serious about your health, that you're not satisfied with the present you, and you're damn well going to do something about it. They can help and they'll only be too happy to do so — for they stand to gain also, with a healthier, more energetic, friendlier and more caring partner, father or colleague.

Now for the initial three steps.

STEP ONE — Check with your doctor

STEP TWO — Check your weight

STEP THREE — Check your measurements — chest, waist and hips

Now you're ready to go.

Soon you'll be waking up in the morning hungry, energetic, and glowing with health. Your self-image and self-control will reflect a new you — and take it from me, it's a marvellous feeling.

But enough of the born-again sermonising — now for the nitty-gritty. Are you ready for the challenge?

HEIGHT/WEIGHT TABLE

ft ins	cms	stones	lbs	kg
5'4"	162.5	8.11 – 10.6	123 – 146	55.8 – 66.3
5'5"	165	9 – 10.10	126 – 150	57.2 – 68
5'6"	167.5	9.4 – 11	130 – 154	59 – 69.9
5'7"	170	9.8 – 11.5	134 – 159	60.8 – 72.1
5'8"	172.5	9.2 – 11.10	138 – 164	62.6 – 74.4
5'9"	175	10.2 – 12	142 – 168	64.4 – 76.2
5'10"	178	10.6 – 12.7	146 – 175	66.3 – 79.4
5'11"	180.5	10.12 – 12.12	150 – 180	68 – 81.6
6'0"	183	11 – 13.2	154 – 184	69.9 – 83.5
6'1"	185.5	11.4 – 13.7	158 – 189	71.7 – 85.7
6'2"	188	11.10 – 13.10	164 – 192	74.4 – 87
6'3"	190.5	12 – 14	168 – 196	76.2 – 88.9
6'4"	193	12.3 – 14.7	171 – 203	77.6 – 92

PROGRESS CHART

It is not necessary to measure yourself on a weekly basis
— once a fortnight will do, and should reveal a marked
difference.

First Week

Weight . . . .

Chest . . . .

Waist . . . .

Hips . . . .

Second Week

Weight . . . .

Chest . . . .

Waist . . . .

Hips . . . .

Third Week

Weight . . . .

Chest . . . .

Waist . . . .

Hips . . . .

Fourth Week

Weight . . . .

Chest . . . .

Waist . . . .

Hips . . . .

Fifth Week

Weight . . . .

Chest . . . .

Waist . . . .

Hips . . . .

Sixth Week

Weight . . . .

Chest . . . .

Waist . . . .

Hips . . . .

Seventh Week

Weight . . . .

Chest . . . .

Waist . . . .

Hips . . . .

Eighth Week

Weight . . . .

Chest . . . .

Waist . . . .

Hips . . . .

PRE-DIET FOOD RECORD

KEEP A RECORD OF EVERYTHING YOU EAT AND
DRINK, INCLUDING SNACKS, AND HOW MUCH
IT WEIGHS.

Date	Breakfast	Snacks

Your weight and vital statistics — before Week 1
of Basic Programme:

Lunch   Dinner

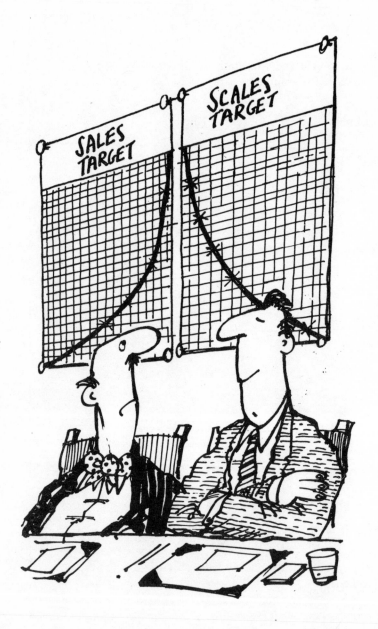

CHAPTER 2

The Basic Weight-Control Programme

First, the bad news. For the next two weeks you're *totally off* the following foods (in fact, some you should say goodbye to for ever more):

Alcohol

Avocados

Bacon

Bananas

Biscuits

Butter

Cakes

Cheese (hard, soft or
   semi-soft)

Chocolates (of any shape,
   type or description)

Cream

Crisps

Dried Fruits

Fish fingers

Jams, jellies and marmalade

Luncheon meats, etc

Milk, full-fat or
   semi-skimmed

Nuts (including peanut
   butter)

Pasta

Pies

Pizza

Potatoes

Rice

Sausages

Sugar

Sweetcorn

Sweets

The good news follows. Here's what you *must have* — in any 24-hour period — at *any time*. You'll probably be surprised at *how much* it is, but you have to eat it *all* by the time you stagger off to bed.

All the weights quoted below in the various sections are actual *eating* weights, what you put into your mouth. Allow for shrinkage and bone content, when cooking meat for instance, so don't cheat yourself. You'll lose the *maximum* amount of weight by eating the *maximum* amount allowed.

FRUIT = 4 servings
FAT = 3 servings
MILK/YOGHURT = ½ pint (285ml) or 5 oz (140g)
CARBOHYDRATE = 2 servings
PROTEIN = 7 servings
VEGETABLES = unlimited
DRINKS = unlimited

FRUIT

4 servings daily

1 serving = 1 orange, apple, pear, peach, medium grapefruit
 or kiwi fruit

or

2 plums, 2 satsumas, 2 tangerines or 3
 clementines

or

3 oz (85 g) grapes

or

5 oz (140g) any berries

or

4 oz (115g) melon

or

4 fl. oz (115ml) *any* unsweetened fruit juice

The only fruit you can eat in unlimited quantities is rhubarb. But be warned. If eaten in excess, it acts as a laxative.

All fruit contains a proportion of natural sugar, but however natural, it's still fattening! So don't fall into the trap of eating unlimited quantities of fruit on the assumption that it doesn't make much of a difference to your weight. It *does*. The four fruit servings you're allowed are ample, but they mean just that — four servings. A serving of two plums doesn't mean a bagful, and

3 oz (85g) grapes doesn't involve plucking them carelessly from the fruit bowl in the course of an evening. (You can, of course, remove the pips and the stalks *before* weighing, but I doubt if you're that desperate.)

I frankly enjoy eating the whole fruit in preference to the juice only (they've also got more fibre). A peeled tangerine in sections, an apple thinly sliced, a peach neatly quartered — they all take much longer to eat and are, therefore, more satisfying. The skin, the pith and the fibre content of whole fruits are all healthy and nutritious, and are a great aid to your food programme. One thing you'll notice very quickly is how marvellous fruits taste now you're eating correctly. Eating will be a much more pleasurable and enjoyable experience. You've probably forgotten how wonderful foods can taste. Take your time and enjoy the experience.

If you're going to use the fruits as eating-any-time food — at the office, in the car, or walking around the house — choose the ones that take the longest to eat: the satsumas, tangerines, oranges and clementines.

When berries are in season (and that's virtually year-round now), they're great value. Five oz (140 g) strawberries is one heck of a bowlful, and if you can't ignore your lust for cream all over them, substitute the natural yoghurt, and sprinkle with a sweetener. Delicious!

Why not try taking grapes off the stalk and open freezing them on a tray? Just like hard sweets, they take a long time to eat so you can keep your mouth full all day (especially if you've given up smoking).

Instead of kidding yourself into believing that only chocolate can give you that instant energy, eat some fruit. It's got that sugar kick, but it's better for your weight, your teeth, and your body.

Lots of exotic fruits have appeared over the last few years, and although I haven't mentioned them specifically, use your common sense. Think of size, so one mango or guava is a serving, two lychees or passion fruit are a serving, etc. (Avoid dates, though, they're virtually pure sugar carbohydrate.)

Rhubarb is the only unlimited fruit. And before you shrug it off as bitter or unpleasant, try it cooked slowly in a small amount of low-calorie blackcurrant squash, Diet Coke or, best of all, low-calorie ginger ale! Add sweetener if desired after cooking. Rhubarb and ginger is a classic combination.

Canned fruits in syrup are a *no-no* (that sugar again), but many supermarkets sell fruits canned or preserved in natural juices.

One tip. Don't go berserk on fruit juices in hot weather. Four fl. oz (115 ml) is the serving, so measure it out initially. Then you'll be able to judge in the future.

Use your allotment of fruits in many different ways for variety and added satisfaction: in yoghurt, in some of your fruit juice, by themselves, in salads, in fruit salads, over cereal, with meat and fish . . .

FAT

3 servings daily

1 serving = l level teaspoon low-fat spread (Gold, Delight or
Outline, or similar products)
or
1 level teaspoon vegetable oil
or
1 level teaspoon vinaigrette (see below), salad
cream or mayonnaise

In your first flush of enthusiasm, you may be thinking that fats are the last thing you should be eating. Not true. You need a certain proportion of fats on a balanced diet, especially for your skin and hair, and you're only allowed 3 teaspoon servings daily because of the fat in the other foods you are allowed to eat, particularly protein. Eating too much fat leads to high levels of cholesterol in the blood, and this is associated with an increased risk of heart disease. Too much fat is − obviously − fattening as well.

This is why in The Businessman's Diet you're not allowed to eat sausages, bacon, canned meats, cream, chocolate, cream and hard cheeses and butter, and have only a limited number of eggs per week (the yolks are quite cholesterol high, but are valuable in this diet). I'm not going into the never-ending debate of butter versus the low-fat spreads. Experience has taught me that low fat spreads have a slight advantage. Use the fat allowance, whatever your choice, for spreading on bread or toast, for cooking (eggs particularly), for pouring melted over your vegetables, or to dress salads.

Salad Dressings

In teaspoon quantities, you can't make much of a salad dressing. The classic vinaigrette is made of four parts oil to one part vinegar, but three to one would be a more sensible alternative for our programme. Always use the polyunsaturated vegetable oils − safflower, sunflower, corn or grapeseed. Make up a vinaigrette in a little screw-top jar, using 3 tablespoons oil (3 teaspoons = 1 tablespoon) and 1 tablespoon vinegar (or lemon juice). Use a multiple of these, for most dressings keep well in the fridge. Because of this dilution, you can reckon on a ½ tablespoon giving you about the 1 teaspoon serving allowed. (That seems a fraction more generous, doesn't it!)

Never forget to season your dressing well, ringing the changes for differing flavours: use salt (lightly), pepper, white or black and freshly ground, some made or grainy mustard or some mustard powder, some curry powder or paste, tomato purée, or even soy or Worcestershire sauce. If you add a little garlic or raw horseradish, you'll have a powerful flavour, but the dressing won't last so long. *Never* add sugar to a dressing.

As far as the mayonnaise and salad dressing are concerned, they can be 'diluted' with a little of your skimmed milk or yoghurt allowance. Merely adding 1 teaspoon of mayonnaise to some natural yoghurt makes a delightful dressing − and it goes much further too! You can spice these up as well in much the same way as the vinaigrette − with garlic, curry powder or paste, Tabasco (go easy), chilli powder or paprika, some chopped onion or herbs. Even natural yoghurt alone with any of these additions (particularly garlic) makes a good dressing.

SKIMMED MILK OR YOGHURT

½ pint (285 ml) skimmed milk daily
or
1 × 5 oz (140 g) carton natural, unsweetened yoghurt daily

Skimmed Milk

If you're as decrepit as I am, you'll probably remember a song popular during the war, 'You'll get used to it' (it might have been sung by George Formby). That's the perfect theme song for skimmed milk. You'll get used to it. And I assure you that once you do, you won't go back to the full-fat variety. I've used skimmed milk for years now, and I can state with my hand on my heart that I can't bear tea, coffee or cereal with full-fat milk – it's far too fatty and rich and leaves an unpleasant coated feeling in my mouth.

I grant you it doesn't have the creamy taste and texture of the full-fat variety. What it does have, however, is all the vitamins and nutrients of its older brother, and a *minute* percentage of the fat content.

And this *does* make a difference. You probably drink six to eight cups of tea or coffee daily – that's about the national average. And if all those cups contain full-fat milk with its full-fat content, you're way over the top of your allowance even before you begin on the food. *And* you've probably put milk over your breakfast cereal or cooked your porridge in milk. Use skimmed milk instead for everything, and the result is weight loss and better health.

FAT IN MILK

Type of Milk	% Fat
Skimmed	Almost 0
Semi-skimmed	2
Full-fat	4

Skimmed milk is available everywhere − from the milkman, in the supermarkets or you can make it up yourself from the powder. My choice is the fresh skimmed milk delivered daily by the milkman. If you're getting it this way, don't let him fob you off with the semi-skimmed variety. Milkmen seem to think that they're lessening your torture by doing it gradually. Insist on skimmed milk and only skimmed milk. Some people prefer the long-life skimmed milk which lasts for an eternity out of the fridge: others prefer to make it up from the powder. One solution to the weakness aspect is to use the correct amount of powder with half the water required: the result is less quantity but a thicker, more visually appealing, and slightly richer, but still skimmed, milk.

Marvel produce packets of low-fat skimmed milk sachets that are ideal for the desk or the briefcase. Each sachet contains enough powder for one cup − roughly one-tenth of your daily allowance. They're small, useful and perfect for your programme. There's absolutely no excuse for drinking tea or coffee with full-fat milk. Order your hot drinks black and add the sachet.

The same applies to those drink machines that lurk in every corner. Press the 'black' button and add the skimmed milk. Simple and effective. And you'll get the bonus of feeling virtuous, while all around you are gaining weight with fatty drinks. You're losing weight and are in control. Give the skimmed milk a good chance to succeed. I can't give you a money-back guarantee that you'll never touch another drop of full-fat milk, but the odds are definitely in your favour. At the worst, 'you'll get used to it.'

Yoghurt

As for yoghurt, the variety on the market is bewildering enough for even the most fastidious shopper. What you're looking for is a low-fat, natural, skimmed-milk yoghurt. Whether it contains fruit or not makes little difference − the amount of fruit content is minimal − but the natural yoghurt is more *useful*. Be on your guard with the full-fat creamy yoghurts over which the Greek variety reigns supreme. Often served abroad with chopped nuts and honey (and in Greek restaurants), it's a great temptation, but you know better than to succumb. Avoid it, along with all the other full-fat or creamy varieties, and stick to your skimmed milk, natural yoghurts. (You could of course make your own low-fat yoghurt at home; individual appliances will give their own instructions.)

Natural yoghurt is incredibly versatile. Use it over cereals instead of skimmed milk for a change, or over fruits, to accompany curries (with chopped cucumber and spices), in salad dressings (see above), with onion and spices in a baked potato (once you're allowed these again, it's a perfect substitute for soured cream), for cooking (chicken and fish are delicious cooked in yoghurt), or with any number of ingredients.

If you're a chocoholic and crave a chocolatey taste (see Chapter Five for some further advice), add a teaspoon of real cocoa powder or carob to the yoghurt. (Carob, in powder or whole kernel form, is available at most health-food shops; it is much more nutritious than chocolate.)

You can get natural fruit flavourings at any supermarket and, at more up-market shops, brandy, wine or liquor essences. Add natural yoghurt with a little brandy essence to strawberries for a superb sweet − exotic, luxurious and highly nutritious. How's that for healthy eating!

Remember, though, that you're allowed *only* ½ pint (285 ml) skimmed milk per day, *or* (not as well as) a 5 oz (140 g) carton of yoghurt. Measure your daily allowance carefully, and stick to it.

CARBOHYDRATE

2 servings daily

1 serving = 1 oz (30 g) bread or cereal

The three forms of carbohydrate are sugars, starches and cellulose or dietary fibre, and they provide energy in calorie form. This is why carbohydrates are often thought to be dietary villains, for those sugar and starch calories not immediately used up by

FIBRE FOODS

Try to eat at least 1 oz (30g) fibre daily.

Bread (1 oz/30 g)

Wholemeal 3g
Brown 1.5g
White 0.9g

Potatoes (3 oz/85 g)

Baked in jacket 3g
Boiled with skin 3g
Boiled without skin 1g

Pasta (3 oz/85 g)

Wholemeal 6g
Ordinary 2g

Rice (3 oz/85 g)

Brown 3g
White 2g

Pulses (1 oz/30 g)

Lentils 4 g
Red Kidney beans 5g

Fruits

Raspberries (5 oz/140 g)
  10.5 g
Blackberries (5 oz/140 g)
  10.5 g
Strawberries (5 oz/140 g)
  3 g
1 medium banana 3 g
1 medium orange 2.5 g

Fruits *(continued)*

1 medium pear 2.4 g
1 medium apple 2 g
1 oz (30 g) raisins 2 g
Cherries (4 oz/115 g)
  1.7 g
1 medium peach 1.4 g
1 medium grapefruit 1 g
Melon (4 oz/115g) 0.7 g
White grapes (3oz/85 g)
  0.7g
Black grapes (3 oz/85g)
  0.2 g

Vegetables (1 4-5 oz/ 115-140 g serving)

Peas 7 g
Spinach 5 g
Broccoli 5 g
Sweetcorn 5 g
Green beans 4 g
Carrots 3 g
Leeks 3 g
Parsnips, Cabbage,
  Mushrooms 2.8 g
Brussels sprouts,
  Swede 2 g
Tomatoes (2 average)
  1.7g
Cauliflower (raw) 1.2g
Lettuce 0.4 g

physical energy, are stored by the body as fat.

Sugars you have already been warned about. The natural sugars of fruit should be taken in the limited quantities suggested. Refined sugars are 'empty' calories (with no nutritional value whatsoever) and should be avoided like the plague (if you still have a sweet tooth, use sweeteners, see page 43).

The starches are present in foods which are usually cooked, which also contain worthwhile nutrients, and thus have a dietary value. These include grains, wheat, oats, rice – in wholemeal bread and breakfast cereals, for instance – and potatoes, pulses and some other vegetables. For the moment, on the basic programme, your carbohydrate intake is limited to breads and cereals.

Cellulose carbohydrates are found in grains, vegetables and fruit and are unable to be digested by humans. Rather than being useless, however, this is the dietary fibre so vital to health. Dietary fibre helps regulate the bowel, preventing constipation, protecting against bowel problems (including cancer of the bowel and diverticulitis), and contains many vitamins and nutrients. Also, most importantly in your weight-control programme, fibre foods take a lot of chewing and eating – and digesting – and therefore fill you up and keep you feeling satisfied for longer. You should try to eat at least 1 oz (30 g) of fibre daily.

Please note that at this stage you get two servings of bread and/or cereal, but that's a *total*: it's one of each or two of either.

Breads

This category includes all types of bread: rolls, baps, crispbreads, crumpets, toasted breads and rolls, Melba toast, bagels, pitta bread, matzoh, water biscuits, muffins, Scotch pancakes and scones. As far as nutrients and fibre are concerned, wholewheat or 'natural' products are superior to refined 'white' breads or cereals.

Please note that 1 oz (30 g) bread is *not* one slice, for all bread (and bread products) weigh differently. Granary bread weighs heavy, while you'll get two slices of Nimble or Slimcea bread to 1 oz (30 g). It's up to you if you prefer quantity or quality. My particular recommendation is the best granary or wholewheat you can find. Try, too, the baked half wholewheat rolls available from any good supermarket: they're crunchy, taste good, transport well, and you get two or three per 1 oz (30 g). They also take a long time to eat, a real plus, for the longer something takes to eat – I cannot repeat this often enough – the more satisfying it is.

The heavier breads like pitta, bagels, crumpets and scones are tempting, admittedly, but when you realise that you only get 2 square inches (5 square cm) of crumpet for your serving, you might settle for quantity rather than superficial attraction! (Some of the sweeter breads contain sugar, too, remember).

Most breads and bread products are sold pre-sliced, and one initial weighing at home is sufficient to get a fix on what you need when you haven't got the scales handy. But slicing your own bread is a whole new ball game. No matter how long you've been weighing your foods, don't delude yourself that you can always judge 1 oz (30g) of bread. *You can't.* Human nature being what it is, every time you slice without weighing, the actual weight increases; somehow it never reduces . . . miraculous, in fact. I fell into this trap some time ago. I'd maintained my weight for a good number of months and was convinced I knew what a 1 oz (30 g) slice looked like. After two months of non-weighing, I attended a monthly meeting of lecturers, and was horrified at my weight: the complacent guru was 6 lb (2.7 kg) over! Ashamed to show my face in decent society, I slunk home and cut a slice of granary bread I had previously judged to be 1 oz (30 g) – 3½ oz (100 g), would you believe? *Never* think you know it all – it's a complacency and unwillingness to face the truth that produces that sometimes unfortunate reflection in the mirror at dawn.

Cereals

You can choose from a vast selection of cereals. They are all acceptable, except for the varieties that are sugar or honey coated – although most have some sugar content. Weights are important here as well, and I'd go for quantity over quality rather than the other way round. An oz (30 g) of Rice Krispies, Puffed

Wheat, or Special K gives you a heaped bowlful, but 1 oz (30 g) of muesli results in a nut and raisin virtually.

My own favourite breakfast cereal is porridge oats, one of the few cereals with no sugar content at all. Soak your measured quantity in skimmed milk overnight to make the oats soften and expand, and become more digestible, and cook slowly in the morning. Add a sprinkle of sweetener when cooked, and eat, hot, sweet and lots of it, with a teaspoon. (I'm sure you realise why I eat porridge with a teaspoon ... it prolongs the pleasure and increases the satisfaction!) It will really stick to your ribs and keep you well satisfied until lunch. You can do the same with proper oatmeal – fine, medium or coarse.

Try your cereals with yoghurt instead of skimmed milk for a change, or accompanied by some of your fruit allowance. An American friend suggests 1 oz (30 g) bran flakes covered with some natural yoghurt, topped with 5 oz (140 g) strawberries, and sprinkled with an artificial sweetener. The result is a cross between a fruity cheesecake and a trifle – an absolute treat for the sweet tooth, and highly nutritious into the bargain.

PROTEIN

7 servings daily

1 serving = 1 oz (30 g) beef, veal, ham, liver, skinless
chicken, turkey or game, or any fish or seafood
or
1 egg (maximum 5 weekly)
or
3 oz (85 g) cottage, curd or Quark-type low-fat
cheese
or
1 oz (30 g) lentils or dried beans

Proteins are required for growth and repair of *all* the organs of the body, and are readily available from meats, fish, eggs and dairy products (milk, cheese, butter, yoghurt, etc) and other sources. The trouble is that many adults in the West are on *too high* a protein intake, and what the body does not use is stored as fat. A large cooked breakfast, an expense-account lunch of steak, and a second protein-rich meal at night, allied to a fairly sedentary life – the lot of the average businessman – means far more protein than is necessary – and indeed, these quantities can be dangerous. Thus we are limited here to 7 oz (200 g) daily.

Meats

Nearly all the meats are acceptable, although the balance is in favour of the *white* meats such as chicken, turkey, rabbit and game birds, as these contain less fat than red meats such as beef. Red meat exceptions are lamb and pork for the time being, but you'll get them back on the menu shortly. Liver and kidneys are also useful protein foods as they contain many nutrients.

When I suggest 5 oz (140g) chicken, I mean 5 oz (140 g) *eating* weight, what you actually put into your mouth. In the case of chicken, which has a high percentage of bone weight and shrinks in the cooking, a gross weight of 9-12 oz (255-340 g) will give you 5-6 oz (140-170 g) net when cooked. You can allow a 4 oz (115 g) shrinkage and bone weight on chops or steaks; which means an 8 oz (225 g) steak gross gives about 4 oz (115g) eating weight.

Cut off and discard the visible fat on all meats. It is the *invisible* fat within the flesh of chops and steaks, etc that melts and comes out – and accounts for the weight loss. Take all skin off chicken and turkey as this contains a lot of fat.

Cook the meat in a way that does not require extra fat. Grilled is the best as the fat drips out and *away* from the flesh. You could also roast, bake or poach, depending on the meat or cut, and there are frying pans in which you can 'dry-fry' meats. Always blot cooked meat on kitchen paper before serving to get rid of the last vestiges of fat.

Fish

All varieties of fish and seafood are acceptable – fresh, frozen, canned or smoked. If canned (salmon, tuna, sardines, etc), avoid those preserved in oil in favour of those in brine, now available everywhere. Smoked salmon, tuna or sardine salad, grilled sole, poached smoked haddock . . . the list is endless, and the world is your oyster (or vice-versa). Do, however, poach, grill or bake your fish rather than frying or deep-frying, or using any cooking method that requires additional fat. Avoid sauces like the plague in this first two-week period.

Eggs

Watch the quantity of eggs — five a week is plenty because of the cholesterol in the yolks — and eat them any way you like: boiling, coddling or poaching saves your fat allowance. For scrambled eggs, use 1 teaspoon low-fat spread and a little skimmed milk, *delicious* with some smoked salmon.

Cheeses

You will have noticed that on the prohibited foods list at the beginning of the chapter are the majority of cheeses, owing to their high fat content. You can, however, have low-fat curd cheese, available at supermarkets and delicatessens, which is made from skimmed milk.

Low-fat curd cheese is less runny than cottage cheese, is easy to spread and very filling. Three oz (85 g) constitutes 1 serving, and mixed with 1 oz (30 g) chopped smoked salmon (also 1 serving) makes a tasty fish pâté for lunch. Spread it on two or three of those pre-baked wholewheat rolls (again about 1 serving) and eat along with the biggest salad you can manage, for a solid, satisfying meal. (Note, please, that you've only eaten *two* of your protein servings, with another five left for dinner. That could be a 5 oz (140 g) steak, 5 oz (140 g) sole, 5 oz (140 g) meat sauce, a quarter-pounder at your favourite hamburger joint, or virtually a half chicken!)

Low-fat Quark-type cheeses are good, and the old stand-by cottage cheese is now sold with various additions such as prawns, cucumber and pineapple. I still prefer the curd cheese, though; it's more filling and spreads without dripping over everything.

After the first two weeks, you will be allowed cheeses other than cottage, curd or low-fat Quark-type. The fat content of cheese ranges enormously from low-fat cottage cheese at one end to Stilton and Lymeswold varieties at the other.

Cheese is a huge temptation. It's always easily available, and we've all been brainwashed to think of dairy foods in any quantity as healthy and essential. This is not quite correct, and you should have a look at the chart below. Prepare, therefore, for your Basic Diet fortnight by clearing your fridge of all the cheeses that you might be tempted to nibble in a moment of weakness. In fact, do the same clear-out with any food that's tempting, easily available, and on your *no-no* list. If they're not there, you can't eat them.

FAT IN CHEESE

Type of Cheese	% Fat
Cottage cheese	4
Low-fat soft cheese (curd)	9
Low-fat hard cheese (Tendale and Shape)	17
Cheese spread	23
Edam type	23
Camembert type	23
Processed cheese	29
Danish Blue	29
Cheddar type	34
Stilton type	40
Lymeswold type	40
Cream cheese	47

VEGETABLES
Unlimited daily

Here's the one category where you can go all the way. There's no limit on quantities you can eat, at any time or of any variety (excepting of course the aforementioned sweetcorn, avocados and potatoes, and pulses which come under protein).

Eat your vegetables raw as a salad, when they are most fibre and vitamin rich, or cook them lightly in a little water or steam them *over* water. Never use fat to cook them if you can help it, although you can put some low-fat spread over them when they're cooked and hot. Try grilling mushrooms instead of frying them in butter; they're delicious. And sprinkling many vegetables with lemon or lime juice gives them a wonderful flavour without any additional fat.

Don't stick to salads of limp lettuce and tired tomatoes. The shops and supermarkets are overflowing with new and exotic vegetables – asparagus, mangetout, fennel, matchstick-thin Kenyan green beans – all of which can be eaten raw or lightly cooked. There is a huge variety of salad leaves available nowadays – endive, chicory, lamb's lettuce, radiccio, oak-leaf lettuce – plus things like cauliflower which are delicious raw.

Use soft, mashed cauliflower as a terrific substitute for potato. Mash it with a little cooked onion, and serve by itself or as a topping for shepherd's or cottage pie. It's hard to tell the difference, and cauliflower is unlimited.

Try shop-prepared salads: there is a wide selection, but avoid those already dressed. Use your own dressing made from a measured amount of vinaigrette, mayonnaise or salad cream (see page 29).

Vegetables don't only arrive in salads or as bridesmaids to meat or fish. A home-made soup with any or all of your favourite veggies should always be on hand at home, or even in the office fridge for enjoying at any time. Eat as many bowls as you want, whenever you want – between meals, at meals, whenever and wherever you feel hungry.

For a soup or vegetable stew, chop up a few onions and at least 1 lb (450 g) of your selected vegetable or vegetables, and 'sweat' them in a little water or stock in a covered pan until soft. Then add more stock or water and blend to a purée. Add flavourings to taste – stock, cubes, curry powder, or any ground spices (cumin or coriander is good with carrot, for instance). Try your soup with the vegetables cut up in it, not blended smooth, to give your eyes as well as your stomach more satisfaction. It will look like a thick stew. Indeed, if you use less stock or water, you can *have* a vegetable stew, either for a hot main course or for an accompanying vegetable dish. Making it in quantities, using all your favourite vegetables, and having it there, ready to eat, is the secret.

If you're buying canned vegetables, look for the varieties without added salt. We all consume far too much salt.

I don't have the space to list all the vegetables you're allowed, but you really can't have too many – so let your imagination and your appetite run riot!

DRINKS

Unlimited daily

Drink anything you like, whenever you like, and in whatever quantity you like, although the obvious exceptions are alcohol and drinks containing sugar. Milk we have already discussed.

Any sort of coffee (instant, decaffeinated, ground, coffee bags) is acceptable, but I suggest you cut down on *black* coffee and tea. Large quantities of either appear to adversely affect the stomach, sleep patterns and nerves. Coffee or tea with some of your skimmed milk allowance is fine, plus any artificial sweetener of your choice. *No sugar*! Tea with lemon is refreshing, and you can ring the changes by including a slice of lime, or by icing the tea and serving it with mint. A pleasant alternative to the normal range of teas are the herbal ones: try rosehip or camomile, or a variety of others. Perhaps I believe the health-food hype, but I do find a cup of rosehip tea quite soothing and relaxing.

If you're looking for a night-time drink, try the new skimmed-milk, artificially-sweetened chocolate powders available at supermarkets and chemists. They generally come in sachets, some flavoured with mint, some with orange. If you're a minor chocoholic, these chocolate drinks will satisfy that craving – partially anyway.

Any quantity of water is OK. A number of spas and health farms, especially abroad, advocate drinking at least 4-5 pints (2.2-2.8 litres) daily. I'm not convinced, however, that quantities like this are desirable, as the possible benefits are negated by the time spent in the loo.

One health suggestion that does make sense is a water purifier.

You can buy a filter jug arrangement at a chemist or health-food store. The biological benefits are a bit obscure, but the difference in taste is remarkable. On balance, they're a good investment.

The list of bottled waters, fizzy or still, is endless, and growing by the day. Half the business community swears by them, but an increasingly vocal minority is equally antagonistic. To be quite frank, the long list of ingredients printed in miniscule type on the labels is incomprehensible to the layman, and, so I've heard, equally baffling to the chemist. Nevertheless, each brand of mineral water has its disciples, so it's really a question of personal taste. My preference is the Italian Pellegrino.

All bottled waters have one virtue in common: they give you that holier-than-thou feeling of moral superiority. 'Aren't I doing well?' That's a real plus. Whether the water promises eternal youth, a cure for housemaid's knee, or a miraculous sexual awakening, whether it's bottled in Surbiton or Transylvania, the bottom line is they're all definitely harmless, possibly beneficial, and generally satisfying.

The last year or so has seen a great increase in the varieties of genuine diet drinks available. What I mean by genuine diet drinks are those that contain no sugar, or sugar *nom-de-plumes* (ie honey, dextrose, glucose, or anything else that ends in *ose*). Avoid the ones that advertise *lower sugar* and *less sugar*. What you want is *no sugar*. Diet Coke and Pepsi have been joined by Diet 7-Up, Tang, Lilt, One-Cal and many others. Most of them are rather sweet, but they do the trick and quench your thirst. Some regular users maintain that they actually increase your desire for sweet drinks so you consume more and more. I believe this is true of a lot of products artificially sweetened, but that remains a problem to be solved by future nutritionists. Meanwhile, try them all. You're sure to find one or two that you find refreshing and pleasant, and they do fill you up.

Natural fruit juices are, of course, acceptable, but they count as fruit servings (you're allowed four fruit servings daily, remember). Fruit juices are, therefore, limited. The alternatives — water, mineral water, tea, coffee, herbal teas, and genuine diet drinks — are unlimited.

SEASONINGS

Take advantage of all the flavouring 'condiments'. These include salt, pepper, herbs, spices, flavourings, stock cubes, certain sauces such as soy and Worcestershire, or any of the artificial sweeteners.

Be careful with salt as we eat far too much, and this can contribute to heart disease and high blood pressure. Always choose foods without salt – cereals or canned foods, for instance – and if your food is cooked with a little salt, that salt shaker on your dining table is totally redundant.

Any of the sweeteners are acceptable, but avoid the ones that contain 50 per cent sugar (yes, they do exist). I've never been able to kick the sweetener habit, although it's my favourite New Year resolution. Some have more of an after-taste than others, but I'm sure you'll find one that suits you – there are dozens of brands on the market.

Although they might appear to be more relevant under the fruit category, the range of 100 per cent fruit jams and marmalades at health-food shops can be viewed as a seasoning – but to be used in very moderate quantities. They contain no sugar or any ingredient that ends in *ose*. I heartily recommend them but they must be kept in the fridge as they contain no preservatives.

BASIC PROGRAMME MENU SUGGESTIONS

During your two-week basic diet you can devise your own daily menus or follow some of the suggestions given on pages 44-57. Eat *all* your allowance in the 24-hour period. Measure your milk and/or yoghurt allowance carefully, dividing it between all the projected uses. For snacks, see page 65.

WEEKDAY 1

Breakfast

    4 fl. oz (115 ml) unsweetened orange juice
    1 oz (30 g) cornflakes, with skimmed milk or yoghurt
    Tea or coffee unlimited – no sugar

Lunch

    3 oz (85 g) smoked salmon
    1 oz (30 g) granary bread, with 1 level teaspoon low-fat
      spread
    4 oz (115 g) fresh fruit salad, with yoghurt if desired
    Tea, coffee, mineral water or diet drink

Dinner

    4 oz (115 g) calf's liver
    Parsnips, carrots, green beans, with 2 level teaspoons
      low-fat spread
    10 oz (285 g) strawberries, with yoghurt if desired
    Coffee, tea or mineral water

'It's absolutely vital to have readily available, ready washed and peeled *any food on which there are* no *restrictions – carrots, celery, or any vegetables – for immediate use in case of emergency!! Avoids the impulsive death wish.'*
                                  Arnold Shuter, Accountant

WEEKDAY 2

Breakfast

1 pink grapefruit

1 poached egg on 2 oz (60 g) granary toast, with 1 level
teaspoon low-fat spread

Plus as many grilled tomatoes and mushrooms as you
want

Tea or coffee unlimited — no sugar

Lunch

3 oz (85 g) cooked, skinless chicken breast

Green beans, broccoli, tomatoes, courgettes

5 oz (140 g) strawberries, with yoghurt if desired

Tea, coffee, mineral water or diet drink

Dinner

3 oz (85 g) grilled Dover sole

Carrots, peas and large mixed salad

Add 2 level teaspoons vinaigrette, salad cream or
mayonnaise to the salad, or 2 level teaspoons low-fat
spread to the hot vegetables

8 oz (225 g) fresh fruit salad, with yoghurt if desired

Coffee, tea or mineral water

WEEKDAY 3

Breakfast

4 oz (115 g) melon
2 oz (60 g) Bran Flakes, with skimmed milk or yoghurt
Tea or coffee unlimited — no sugar

Lunch

3 oz (85 g) grilled turbot
Asparagus and/or a large salad, with 2 level teaspoons
   low-fat spread
1 kiwi fruit
Tea, coffee, diet drink or mineral water

Dinner

1 grapefruit
4 oz (115 g) grilled fillet steak
Peas, beans, tomatoes, mushrooms with 1 level
   teaspoon low-fat spread
4 oz (115 g) fresh fruit salad, with yoghurt if desired
Coffee, tea or diet drink

WEEKDAY 4

Breakfast

2 oz (60 g) Cornflakes, with 5 oz (140 g) raspberries,
and skimmed milk or yoghurt
Tea and coffee unlimited — no sugar

Lunch

3 oz (85 g) lean roast beef
Brussels sprouts, parsnips, beans
4 oz (115 g) fresh fruit salad, with yoghurt if desired
Coffee, tea or mineral water

Dinner

1 large bowl home-made vegetable soup
4 oz (115 g) baked or grilled monkfish (anglerfish)
Mixed green salad, with 3 teaspoons mayonnaise,
vinaigrette or salad cream
1 kiwi fruit
Coffee, lemon tea or mineral water

*'The best incentive to succeed is to make it hurt —
somehow. I made it very public and kept myself aware
that everyone knew I was trying to slim. I also told them
what it cost me to do the course, which helped me to
remember my failure was going to be a story against my
own pride.'*

Michael Hammond, JP, Managing Director
Hammonds AV-VIDEO Services

WEEKDAY 5

Breakfast

4 fl. oz (115 ml) unsweetened apple juice
1 oz (30 g) Rice Krispies, with yoghurt or skimmed milk
Tea or coffee unlimited — no sugar

Lunch

3 oz (85 g) plainly cooked game (pheasant, quail,
   pigeon, rabbit, venison — no extras!)
Carrots, beans, cauliflower, with 1 teaspoon low-fat
   spread
5 oz (140 g) raspberries, with yoghurt if desired
Coffee, tea, diet drink or mineral water

Dinner

4 oz (115 g) fresh fruit salad
4 oz (115 g) shrimps, with large mixed salad and 1 level
   teaspoon dressing of choice
1 oz (30 g) granary bread, with 2 level teaspoons low-fat
   spread
3 oz (85 g) grapes
Coffee, tea or mineral water

WEEKEND 1

Breakfast

2 whole tangerines, in sections
1 oz (30 g) Bran Buds, with skimmed milk or yoghurt
Tea or coffee unlimited — no sugar

Lunch

Quarter-pounder at your favourite hamburger joint, in a 1
oz (30 g) bun. (This will contain a certain amount of
fat, so you're cut down to only 1 teaspoon fat today —
and definitely *no* French fries or milk shake!)
Tea, coffee, or diet drink

Dinner

4 oz (115 g) melon
3 oz (85 g) ham steak
Parsnips, carrots, broccoli, courgettes, with 1 teaspoon
low-fat spread
8 oz (225 g) fresh fruit salad, with yoghurt if desired
Coffee, tea or diet drink

*'The easiest way to lose weight is to get your wife to go on
a diet, then she won't cook anything fattening!'*
N.L., Professional Engineer

WEEKEND 2

For early-morning 'munchies', eat an apple. Cut it in four, core it, and eat slowly.

Brunch

4 oz (115 g) melon

2-egg omelette, made with 1 level teaspoon low-fat
   spread

Plus as many grilled tomatoes and mushrooms as you
   can eat

2 oz (60 g) granary toast, with 1 level teaspoon low-fat
   spread

Tea or coffee unlimited – no sugar

Dinner

5 oz (140 g) roast veal

Peas, carrots, cauliflower, with 1 level teaspoon low-fat
   spread

4 oz (115 g) fresh fruit salad. Add 1 kiwi fruit, cover with
   yoghurt, and sprinkle with sweetener if desired

Coffee, tea or mineral water

'Just as a dry alcoholic is still an alcoholic, a slim fatty is one binge away from perdition.'
   Eden Phillips, Journalist and Publishing Executive

WEEKDAY 6

Breakfast

1 grapefruit
2 oz (60 g) Cornflakes, with skimmed milk or yoghurt
Tea or coffee unlimited — no sugar

Lunch

Asparagus to start (as much as you like — enjoy
  yourself), with 3 level teaspoons low-fat spread
3 oz (85 g) fresh poached or grilled salmon
Peas, carrots, spinach
5 oz (140 g) raspberries, with yoghurt if desired
Tea, coffee or mineral water

Dinner

1 huge bowl home-made vegetable soup
4 oz (115 g) cooked, skinless chicken
Parsnips, green beans, carrots, courgettes, with some
  lemon or lime juice sprinkled over them
2 peaches
Coffee, tea or diet drink

*'Try to increase the exercise. I walk to the tube station
(approximately 15 minutes) nearly every morning.'*
                              Richard Pain, Solicitor

WEEKDAY 7

Breakfast

4 fl. oz (115 ml) unsweetened grapefruit juice
1 poached egg on 2 oz (60 g) granary toast, with 2 level
   teaspoons low-fat spread
Plus as many grilled tomatoes and mushrooms as you
   want
Tea or coffee unlimited — no sugar

Lunch

3 oz (85 g) lean roast beef, with horseradish sauce (not
   too much)
Parsnips, carrots, green beans
4 oz (115 g) fresh fruit salad, with yoghurt if desired
Tea, coffee or mineral water

Dinner

4 oz (115 g) melon
3 oz (85 g) grilled trout
Peas, green beans, with 1 level teaspoon low-fat spread
1 orange or apple
Coffee, tea or mineral water

'I don't have a weight problem because I worry!'
Michael Parkinson, Entertainer

WEEKDAY 8

Breakfast

2 oz (60 g) Bran Flakes, with skimmed milk or yoghurt
3 oz (85 g) grapes
Tea or coffee unlimited — no sugar

Lunch

3 oz (85 g) grilled Dover sole
Mixed green salad, with 2 level teaspoons vinaigrette
1 kiwi fruit
Coffee, tea or diet drink

Dinner

1 grapefruit
4 oz (115 g) calf's liver (try it Italian-style, grilled with
    rosemary and other herbs)
Peas, carrots, green beans, with 1 level teaspoon low-fat
    spread
1 peach
Coffee, tea or mineral water

*'The secret to all diets is regular accountability. Weekly
weighing is the only system that works for me. If these are
missed, then the weight loss process is less effective.'*

Tony Aplin, Chairman, APA

WEEKDAY 9

Breakfast

4 fl. oz (115 ml) unsweetened orange juice

1 oz (30 g) porridge (weighed *dry*, see page 36 for how to prepare), with skimmed milk and sweetener if desired

Tea or coffee unlimited — no sugar

Lunch

4 oz (115 g) melon

4 oz (115 g) tuna fish, with a large mixed salad

1 oz (30 g) granary bread, with 1 level teaspoon low-fat spread

Coffee, tea or mineral water

Dinner

3 oz (85 g) roast veal

Green beans, carrots, broccoli, with 2 level teaspoons low-fat spread

8 oz (225 g) fresh fruit salad, with yoghurt and sweetener if desired

Coffee, tea or diet drink

'I have always been 11 stone — about 5 pounds over-weight. It's caused by sitting slumped watching TV. Recently I did a show in the West End and lost 8 pounds in 10 weeks — through stress, panic and hard work. *So if you want to lose weight . . .'*

Ernie Wise, Entertainer

WEEKDAY 10

Breakfast

1 oz (30 g) Bran Flakes, with 1 sliced medium peach,
    and skimmed milk or yoghurt
Tea or coffee unlimited — no sugar

Lunch

3 oz (85 g) smoked salmon
1 oz (30 g) granary bread, with 1 level teaspoon low-fat
    spread
5 oz (140 g) strawberries, with yoghurt if desired
Coffee, tea or mineral water

Dinner

Asparagus, with 2 level teaspoons low-fat spread
4 oz (115 g) cooked, skinless turkey
Swedes, carrots, peas
1 kiwi fruit and 3 oz (85 g) grapes
Coffee, tea or mineral water

WEEKEND 3

Breakfast

2 clementines
2 poached eggs, on 2 oz (60 g) granary toast, with 2
    level teaspoons low-fat spread
Plus as many grilled mushrooms and tomatoes as you
    can eat
Tea or coffee unlimited — no sugar

Lunch

3 oz (85 g) curd cheese (add a little Marmite for a great
    taste), plus an enormous mixed salad
Cooked rhubarb and apple (use 1 apple and unlimited
    rhubarb, and see page 27)
Coffee, tea or diet drink

Dinner

4 oz (115 g) melon
4 oz (115 g) grilled steak
Parsnips, peas, carrots, Brussels sprouts, with 1 level
    teaspoon low-fat spread
4 oz (115 g) fresh fruit salad
Coffee, tea or mineral water

*'If we took more care of body tone and definition, we
would not only look better, but feel better. Skinny flab is no
more attractive than fat flab!'*
                        — David Quilter, Actor and Jogger

WEEKEND 4

Brunch

5 oz (140 g) strawberries, with yoghurt and sprinkled with sweetener if desired

2 scrambled eggs, made with 1 level teaspoon low-fat spread

Plus as many grilled tomatoes and mushrooms as you want

2 oz (60g) granary toast, with 1 level teaspoon low-fat spread

Tea or coffee, unlimited – no sugar

Dinner

4 oz (115 g) melon

5 oz (140 g) white fish

Asparagus, green beans, carrots, with 1 level teaspoon low-fat spread

6 oz (170 g) grapes

Coffee, tea or diet drink

'I believe the will to see one's life carry on is the greatest spur – another is ambition to attract other people by one's own personal appearance.'

Michael Hammond, JP, Managing Director,
Hammonds AV-VIDEO Services

BASIC PROGRAMME FOOD DIARY

1st Week

Write down the 'limited' food you eat during the day and tick off your servings allowance accordingly.
Unlimited vegetables and drinks – but check exceptions.

Day	Morning	Afternoon	Evening	Servings Allowance
1				4 fruits 3 fats milk/yoghurt 7 protein 2 carbohydrates
2				4 fruits 3 fats milk/yoghurt 7 protein 2 carbohydrates
3				4 fruits 3 fats milk/yoghurt 7 protein 2 carbohydrates

58

4			4 fruits 3 fats milk/yoghurt 7 protein 2 carbohydrates
5			4 fruits 3 fats milk/yoghurt 7 protein 2 carbohydrates
6			4 fruits 3 fats milk/yoghurt 7 protein 2 carbohydrates
7			4 fruits 3 fats milk/yoghurt 7 protein 2 carbohydrates

Weight after Week One on Basic Programme . . . .

BASIC PROGRAMME FOOD DIARY
2nd Week

Write down the 'limited' food you eat during the day and tick off your servings allowance accordingly.
Unlimited vegetables and drinks – but check exceptions.

Day	Morning	Afternoon	Evening	Servings Allowance	
1				4 fruits 3 fats milk/yoghurt 7 protein 2 carbohydrates	☐☐☐☐ ☐☐☐ ☐☐ ☐ ☐☐☐ ☐☐
2				4 fruits 3 fats milk/yoghurt 7 protein 2 carbohydrates	☐☐☐☐ ☐☐☐ ☐☐ ☐ ☐☐☐ ☐☐
3				4 fruits 3 fats milk/yoghurt 7 protein 2 carbohydrates	☐☐☐☐ ☐☐☐ ☐☐ ☐ ☐☐☐ ☐☐

Day	Food groups	Portions
4	4 fruits 3 fats milk/yoghurt 7 protein 2 carbohydrates	☐☐☐ ☐☐ ☐☐ ☐☐ ☐ ☐ ☐☐ ☐☐☐ ☐ ☐
5	4 fruits 3 fats milk/yoghurt 7 protein 2 carbohydrates	☐☐☐ ☐☐ ☐☐ ☐☐ ☐ ☐ ☐☐ ☐☐☐ ☐ ☐
6	4 fruits 3 fats milk/yoghurt 7 protein 2 carbohydrates	☐☐☐ ☐☐ ☐☐ ☐☐ ☐ ☐ ☐☐ ☐☐☐ ☐ ☐
7	4 fruits 3 fats milk/yoghurt 7 protein 2 carbohydrates	☐☐☐ ☐☐ ☐☐ ☐☐ ☐ ☐ ☐☐ ☐☐☐ ☐ ☐

Weight after Week Two on Basic Programme . . . .

61

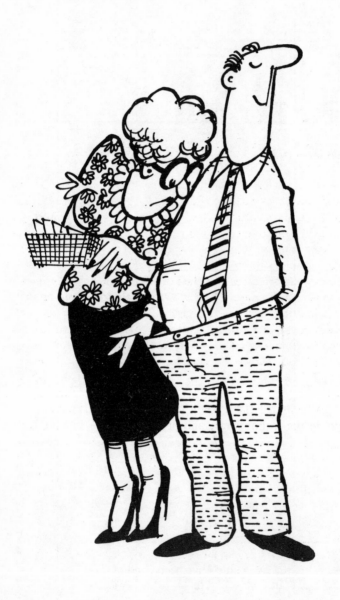

CHAPTER 3

The First Two Weeks:
Progress and Potential Problems

Now that you know what you can and can't eat and drink you must chart your weight losses and fluctuations. Only by noting these can you come to understand your own particular attitudes, and difficult times and situations, and amend them accordingly.

There's certainly no need for an elaborate or complex diary noting every cup of coffee and glass of water, but a weekly sheet similar to the one on pages 58-59 is a great help for, if put on the spot, very few of us can recall what we ate for lunch yesterday, let alone a few days ago. Only the limited foods need be noted – the proteins, fruits, carbohydrates and fats. Forget about the unlimited foods and drinks – vegetables and teas, coffees, mineral waters etc.

Filling in a food and drink diary at *any* time is a real eye-opener, not only for the amount of food that you *over*-eat – generally in the carbohydrate and protein areas – but for the *under*-eating of other foods, especially fruit and vegetables. It's more than likely, therefore that you're actually not eating enough of the correct foods and over-eating the incorrect ones. You'll have realised this, having filled in your *pre*-diet chart.

Note the weights carefully on your chart, and please realise that you're kidding yourself when you write in 'ham sandwich' or 'Sole Meunière': the former could have contained anything from 2-6 oz (60-170 g) ham, and the bread might have been equally light or heavy; the sole could have been fried in *three* times your fat allowance. If you know you've overdone it in one category – you've had too much meat that day, say – don't cut down on the bread or cereal. You can't switch around. Every category has its required quantities, and you'll do best by sticking to them. But I'd prefer you to err on the side of excess and not to cut out or down on any particular category. You're following a balanced food programme, and everything on it is necessary for success.

I fully realise that you don't carry a weighing scale in your brief-case, but an initial weighing at home of certain foods will give you a good basis on which to operate. Meat and fish, for instance, are generally served in 4-6 oz (115-170g) 'eating weight' portions in most restaurants — which is just right — and a good granary bread slice weighs well over 1 oz (30 g). Fruit portions are virtually self-explanatory. Concentrate, therefore, on the breads and proteins; that's often where the danger lies. Keep within the limit, and don't cheat yourself by going below it. You won't lose any more weight by under-eating — it's as great a danger as over-eating. But don't at the same time become obsessive about weighing. Some fanatic followers have been known to go to any lengths to get the correct eating weight — removing the pips from grapes, and taking advantage of the fact that toast weighs less than bread!

EATING IN THE OFFICE

Teas and coffees from the tea lady are no problem. Order them black and add your own skimmed milk. Skimmed milk powder or even fresh skimmed milk can be kept in your office and used regularly. After a few weeks, you soon get used to the taste — and, yes, it *does* make a difference. As I've said, when you total the amount of teas and coffees you have during a working week, it adds up to an enormous amount of weight-producing fats you could well do without. So it's skimmed milk always and whenever.

The same goes for the automatic vending machines. Press the 'black' tea or coffee button, and avoid the hot chocolate one — it's pre-sugared. (And no remarks about how they all taste the same anyway!)

Elevenses and tea-time at your desk can be difficult. If you're locked in to a croissant at 11 am and a bun at tea, *substitution* is the answer: an orange or apple, a couple of tangerines, a bunch of grapes, or the fruit that you'd planned to have for breakfast or for lunch. But it doesn't have to be fruit from your daily four servings; it could be a wholewheat roll, a piece of bread, salad or a soup, the latter not as far-fetched as you might think. Made at home (see page 40), and brought to the office in a thermos flask, it has the enormous advantage of being in unlimited quantities. You *can* send out for soup from the local deli, but it doesn't compare to the home-made variety for flavour, quantity and freshness; and it probably won't meet the requirements of your programme.

Don't work on the off-chance that when 11 o'clock comes around you'll simply ignore the signals from both your brain and your stomach. Don't be a martyr and endure the suffering with pained indifference. If you're hungry at 11 am, *eat* at 11 am. But eat something you're allowed and something that you planned for. Your aim is not so much eliminating the need for a snack at these times, but channelling your need to a snack that you're *allowed*. I referred before to a 'locked-in' habit, and that's exactly the right description. You're 'locked in' to eating at these times. You've done it for years, and there's nothing terrible about it. Just remember that you have a great quantity of foods that you must eat during the 24 hours, but it doesn't have to be eaten at special times of the day, or even in three regular meals.

Meals in the office should present no problem if you've done your homework. Sandwich bars, delis and health-food shops offer an unlimited variety of take-away foods, which will be suitable, but always watch out for over-enthusiastic dressings on salads. Chicken, ham, chopped liver, smoked salmon, tuna or prawn, curd or cottage cheese – in sandwiches (re-plan your carbohydrate intake), or in salads. You can always ask for sandwiches without butter if necessary.

If you know what you're going to be eating at your desk on Thursday, you will have done your scheduling earlier in the week not just for Thursday lunch, but for Thursday breakfast and Thursday dinner as well. You're on a 24-hour schedule. However, if lunch at your desk is a last-minute affair and you haven't had a chance to plan, stick to chicken, prawn and ham salad take-aways, plus soup and fresh fruit.

One client of mine follows a regime of one enormous meal daily. He can't manage breakfast – never could – and generally works *through* lunchtime at his desk – *never* eating in the office – and arrives home around 7 pm for dinner at 8. And that dinner entails all the fruit, proteins, fats, carbohydrates and vegetables that are required. He actually survives the day on numerous cups of coffee with skimmed milk plus a couple of oranges. His wife is totally conversant with his food programme and his PA equally aware. Business lunches are scheduled into his weekly routine and are accounted for correctly. The result? He's lost 35 lbs (15.75 kg) and is maintaining his weight loss.

Maybe it's not a routine you could follow. I certainly couldn't. If I haven't eaten a full breakfast by 7.30 am, I'm as grouchy as a bear for the rest of the day. But it's great for him. Because he's made the programme work around him and work for him. But I frankly would rarely advocate this sort of concentrated eating over a long working day. I believe that your body is a motor, and it needs to be moderately treated with regular servicing and injections of petrol, oil and grease. However, to each his own, and that particular programme works for him. But he plans and consults continually, and that's the answer. Consultation and planning. In Chapter 6 I suggest some business menus for the basic and the bonus diet programmes. You may find them helpful.

Another office hazard would appear to be the 'chocolate run' twice daily. This consists of a junior member of staff taking orders for chocolates and sweets from various executives and delivering them minutes later. You can plead temporary insanity, you can cite medical reasons, you can admit to joining Choco-holics Anonymous (such a group does exist), or can even tell the truth as a last resort. But *stop immediately*. Not only does the chocolate give you a temporary false high, it decays your teeth and makes you fat.

WHEN TO WEIGH AND MEASURE YOURSELF

The most optimistic time to weigh yourself is in the morning after the loo and after a shower. Yes, you do weigh less in the morning than at night – as much as 4 lb (1.8 kg) in some cases – and, a hot bath makes little difference.

You're most likely at your heaviest weight at 8 pm – oddly enough, the time when most slimming clubs meet – and clothes can make a difference. Jeans, for instance, can weight up to 2 lbs (900 g). I find it amusing how incredibly obsessive people can get about weighing in public, choosing what to take off. Removing watches, jewellery, belts and jackets is commonplace, and I recall, with horror, a lady who used to arrive at the class with a friend who accompanied her to the loo. There she would remove her skirt and top, give them to her friend, who would, in turn get them weighed by me. Her friend would then return the clothes to the girl in the loo, who would weigh herself and get the weight of the clothes deducted from the total. And then there was the lady who returned monthly for her weighing in the original dress she'd worn at the group in the early 60s. She'd lost the weight in it and it was her 'lucky frock'.

(Before we turn to each other chuckling manfully about the ladies' obsession with their weights, I must confess that I dressed in a particular way when I was weighed – light trousers, no tie, and short-sleeved shirt! Forgive me, but you can get obsessive, and it's something to be avoided at all costs!)

The best scales to use are the medical scales, with moveable weights, generally found at health centres or doctors' surgeries or, possibly, in the medical room of your office. The scales most usually used, though, are spring scales, which vary considerably. This is the type favoured by the overweight because they get to know exactly where to stand on it to get the answer they want. (And if you really want to get the best result, try a spring scale on a different surface – you'll generally weigh more with the scale on carpet, less on tile and flooring!)

It really doesn't matter when, where or how you weigh

yourself, but always do it on the same scale at the same time, in the same place, and in the same state of undress. I also strongly advise you to weigh yourself weekly. It's not for pure whim that slimming groups weigh at weekly intervals. Daily weighing for the overweight is not only unrealistic, but it can become a source of emotional ups and downs that will be dispiriting and counter-productive.

You step on to the scales – 'Great, I've lost 2 pounds!' Later in the day, you feel that a small eclair or glass of wine is due to you as a reward – what the hell, you did lose 2 pounds. Or, alternatively, you step on to the scales, and 'My God, I've *gained* a pound!' Panic, shock-horror, depression and loss of self-image . . . 'I must be a real pig – this diet doesn't suit me, so to hell with it', or, even worse, 'Today I'm going to cut down to make up for that pound – no lunch, and just a yoghurt for dinner.'

Catch 22 – you can't win. Maybe you can handle the daily variations – and there *will* be such variations daily, sometimes totally inexplicable.

Some claim that they can put on 5 lb (2.25 kg) on a weekend; others believe that over-eating on a particular day takes two weeks to show on the scale. I've yet to get an answer to the question, 'When will that half bottle of wine show?' I sure don't know, and I'm not sure anyone does. One thing I *do* believe is that too much weighing leads to depression, over-elation and obsession – and compulsive weighing is a warning signal of the anorexic.

Measuring yourself every fortnight (more often is narcissistic) is reassuring and beneficial. Unless you're a candidate for the Mr Universe title, confine yourself to chest, waist and hips. Do so naked at the same time as you weigh yourself.

Women generally lose from north to south: first the neck and bust, then the waist, and finally, the most difficult and southerly, hips, thighs and bottom. Men generally lose initially on the tummy and then the chest and hips. And, no, it's not always entirely due to over-indulgence in beer that results in that ugly gut, although it does play an important role.

Keep a note of those measurements every fortnight, and you'll occasionally realise that some weeks you'll lose inches rather than pounds. This means that your body is being realigned.

It's wonderful that you're starting your diet with enthusiasm – and I do understand that you want to chart your progress and see results. But remember – you're not on any miracle pill, and the eating habits of a lifetime won't be changed in two weeks. Chart your progress – fine. But as I've said, weigh yourself once-weekly on the same scale, in the same room, on the same surface and in the same state of undress. May I suggest a Monday morning? It will take you back to schooldays and those terrible Sunday nights when you realised that Monday morning was looming and you hadn't done your homework. It rather calmed the excesses of the weekend, didn't it?

WEIGHT LOSS ON THE BASIC PROGRAMME

It's the obvious question, and one I cannot answer for equally obvious reasons. How much overweight were you? How conscientious have you been on the programme? Have you over-eaten or, equally important, *under*-eaten? Have you skipped categories like fats or skimmed milk? Have you indulged in the odd chocolate bar or biscuit, eating it quickly so it won't be noticed? Or have you starved yourself for a day or two on the mistaken assumption that it will 'speed things up'?

All I can quote are my experiences with clients over the years, experiences which have shattered a few myths that I had previously engraved in stone.

Myths

★ You don't always lose more weight in the first two weeks than someone who has less to lose.

★ You don't always lose less in the first two weeks if you're older.

★ Bone structure (whether you're a light, medium or heavy frame) appears to make little difference in the amount of initial weight loss.

★ Heredity − 'We come from a big-boned family' − seems to make little difference.

★ Men don't lose more weight more quickly than women *pro rata*.

Some beliefs do hold water, however.

Truths

★ You do lose the most weight in the initial fortnight − that is, on a weekly basis.

★ You do suffer from minor headaches, especially if you've previously been somewhat chocoholic and/or eaten lots of sweet and sugary foods. These headaches generally disappear after ten days.

★ A regular exercise routine plays a very substantial part in a successful weight-control programme. I stress the word *regular*, as a once-weekly five-mile jog is counter-productive. Exercise without a proper eating programme is only partly effective, and the same applies in the reverse. Together, they're unbeatable (see Chapter 7).

★ You do weigh more at night than in the morning − at 8 pm you'll weigh your maximum.

★ Constipation, flatulence and diarrhoea occasionally occur on a temporary basis.

★ Cutting out completely − as opposed to cutting down − is more effective in the short and long term regarding the *no-nos* (alcohol, sweets, cakes, etc).

The bottom line of all this is that if you've lost over 7 lb (3 kg) in the first fortnight, you're well on the way to success. If you've lost more, wonderful.

If you've lost less, there is absolutely no reason whatsoever to be depressed. A substantial minority of men lose less initially, but go on to lose steadily over the subsequent weeks and reach their target. Take a good look at your charts. Note your lapses and correct them. Maybe if you hadn't skipped lunch last Tuesday you would have lost more. Perhaps you've forgotten to note that glass of wine with a colleague or maybe you've eaten too much bread. Let me reiterate a previous commandment. *You'll lose the maximum weight by eating the maximum allowed.*

Your weight loss in the first two weeks is important and significant. What is even more important and satisfying is that you know that you're meeting the challenge you've set yourself, and you're succeeding. At this stage, the major changes you've made in your eating programme are a much greater achievement than any weight loss, excellent though that weight loss is.

Congratulations all round − to you certainly, and also to your partners at home and at business who have contributed so much.

AFTER TWO WEEKS

The worst part is over − you've charted your food intake, and you've weighed and measured yourself. You've lost X pounds and you're feeling and looking good. The one thing, though, that you can't expect is immediate universal recognition for your dedication. Perhaps you've gone on diets before, and it's all a bit of a bore to your colleagues; perhaps a number of them feel more than a bit guilty at your success and react by ignoring it; perhaps your family is wary of praise in case you'll feel complacent and kid yourself that 'you've lost enough for the moment'.

Maybe I'm too cynical, and the plain truth is that the loss of 5 lb or even 10 lb (2.25 or 4.5 kg) is not too apparent in two weeks. But *you* know you've lost and the scales show you've lost − as does the tape measure. And that's success in any man's book.

You're now, however, at a very crucial and difficult stage in your programme. You've lost weight, you've lost inches; you've sacrificed food and drink that you like; and you've felt bereft, perhaps even a social outcast at some social occasions. You have an overwhelming feeling of 'What the hell, that's enough for the time being. I'll start dieting again on Monday and celebrate the weight-ioss this week-end.' This is *dangerous*.

Maybe you feel like Andy Cappuccinni, Head of Trading at Smith Barney: 'After I go on a diet for four or so days, I drop a few pounds, lose heart, and then the cycle starts once more – kidding myself until my new clothes are too tight again.' But don't lose heart. If that bulge around the gut is down by 2 inches (5 cm), and you've made a new notch on your trouser belt, you're on the way and doing well. It can only continue, as long as you persevere.

While partners, family and colleagues are genuinely concerned and will try their best to help and co-operate, don't expect the moon. Over the years I have counselled thousands of dieters and have evolved a theory which I call the Jack Sprat Syndrome. You probably know the nursery rhyme: 'Jack Sprat would eat no fat, His wife would eat no lean'. I have come to the conclusion that a high percentage of dieters have slim partners. This can, and does, lead to a good many problems, the basic one being that a person who has never experienced a weight problem of his or her own can never understand yours. What can they know of the pressures and temptations, and of the miseries you experience? Some of them have been brain-washed into believing that it's easy to lose weight – 'simply eat less,' or 'just push yourself away from the table'. Great, they can flaunt an ability to leave food on their plate. Not me, and probably not you either. We finish everything on our plate and, if given the chance, on everybody else's plate also. Be patient and keep consulting. The help and sympathy is there and it's of immense value to your success.

Perhaps you lost some weight even with lapses. Have you reckoned what you could have lost *without* them? It's a salutary exercise.

Re-read your basic programme – your charts – see where you over-ate and, equally as important, where you under-ate. Spot when you binged and when you forgot. Once you can pin-point times and situations, you can prepare. Fore-armed is fore- warned.

Common times of temptation are mid-morning at the office as mentioned above, after-office socialising (the demon drink of course, plus the peanuts and crisps), arriving home in the evening (the welcoming G & T, and the over-long wait for dinner), and the weekend temptations of golf-club bars, Sunday morning fry-ups and dinner at your favourite French restaurant.

If you recognise where the dangers lie, expect them and prepare for them. You don't go into an important meeting without the answers to any possible confrontations with the Board. You use every available bit of information technology to ensure that your forecasts and plans have the greatest chance of success. Do the same with yourself. Your health and your fitness are surely worth the same consideration and foresight.

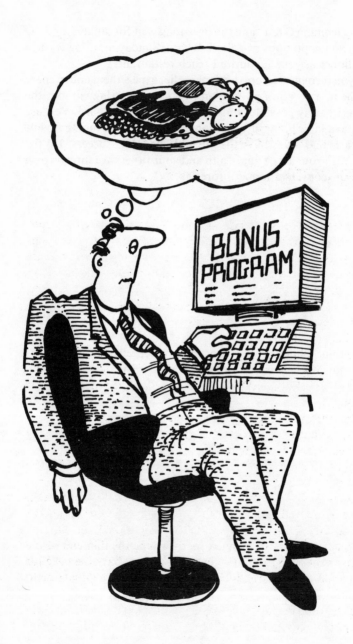

CHAPTER FOUR

The Bonus Weight-Control Programme

The first two weeks are over. You've had difficulties and problems aplenty. You've charted up your foods and drinks, your danger days and hours of those days, and where and when social or business situations have presented temptations. The problems won't go away, that's for sure. But you're far better equipped now to spot them and overcome them. It's *always* difficult to change any basic aspect of your lifestyle, and eating is a vital ingredient of that lifestyle.

Continue planning and consulting, keep charting your progress and continue maintaining your diary. The more you know about yourself, the less you'll deviate and the greater your success.

I did warn you that the first two weeks are the most difficult. Perhaps you need more than a clap on the back and a cheery cry of 'Well done!' It's now time for virtue to be its own reward. Some of the previous *no-no* foods are now allowed in the quantities stated, and new delights are introduced.

However, you must be careful still. You might believe that you're doing well enough on the present programme and don't want to take a chance of putting the weight back on. Or that introducing previously banned foods will be the thin end of the wedge on the road to sin. Or that once you get back the taste for pasta or potatoes, claret or champagne, it will be the final step to binge time.

But before you turn away with righteous indignation, take a look at your chart. Where have you changed your food habits?

Where have you reduced the quantities or resisted those many temptations successfully? Consider the facts. Perhaps you've lost the taste for all that cheese you used to nibble, and could well do without it. Good. But maybe you realise that once you start on rice dishes at the local Indian restaurant you can't stop. If the latter is the case, forget about the extras and the bonuses. Continue the programme you're on.

The basic programme must still be the framework upon which you operate, and to remind you, this is:

FRUIT	= 4 servings
FAT	= 3 servings
MILK/YOGHURT	= ½ pint (285 ml)
	or 5 oz (140 g)
CARBOHYDRATE	= 2 servings
PROTEIN	= 7 servings
VEGETABLES	= unlimited
DRINKS	= unlimited

However, to vary it a little because you've done so well, the ban is now lifted on certain foods.

FRUIT

4 servings daily

As before, but now you can add bananas and dried fruit.

1 serving = 1 medium banana
           or
           1 oz (30g) dried fruit

Both bananas and dried fruit are high in calories which is why they've been omitted until now, but both are full of nutrients. Try cooking the sliced banana with your porridge — it's delicious — or mix some chopped apricots or raisins etc into your cereal.

FAT

3 servings daily

These remain the same.

SKIMMED MILK OR YOGHURT

½ pint (285 ml) or 5 oz (140 g) daily

These, too, remain the same.

CARBOHYDRATE

2 servings daily

As before, but now you can add potatoes, rice and pasta.

    1 serving = 3 oz (85 g) cooked potato
                or
                3 oz (85 g) cooked rice (1 oz/30 g dry)
                or
                3 oz (85 g) cooked pasta (1 oz/30 g dry)

Cook the potatoes in fat-free ways obviously − boiled, steamed or baked. Scrub them clean rather than peeling them, or peel *after* cooking, as most of the nutrients and dietary fibre are in or near the skin. Top baked potatoes with some of your yoghurt allowance mixed with spices and chopped onions/chives/spring onions/garlic to taste. Boil or steam potatoes with herbs − what could be nicer than some tiny Jersey potatoes cooked with some mint? Amplify a potato serving or cottage pie topping with mashed cauliflower as described on page 40, or with cooked mashed celeriac − a classic French combination.

Cooking rice or pasta is plain sailing, but in both cases brown or wholemeal varieties are better for you in terms of nutrients and fibre.

PROTEIN

7 servings daily

As before, but now you can add lamb and pork, and other cheeses.

> 1 serving = 1 oz (30 g) lamb or pork
> or
> 1 oz (30 g) cheese of any type (soft, semi-soft or hard)

With the meat, cook as before in fat-free ways (see page 37) and be sure to cut off all the visible fat.

Be careful with the cheese, particularly Stilton and Lymeswold types (see the chart on page 39), and the *maximum* of cheese allowed is 6 oz (170 g) weekly.

VEGETABLES

Unlimited daily

As before, but now you can add sweetcorn in a limited quantity. It's very high in dietary fibre.

> 1 serving = 3 oz (85 g) sweetcorn

DRINKS

Unlimited daily

As before, but see below.

BONUSES

Now for the bonuses (*boni*?) if you can handle them. These are to be used and enjoyed as required and *if* required. It's not a question of 'Whoopee, school's out!' and into booze and icecream, but a possible increase in the quantities and variety.

Treat the bonuses as you will — as a necessity for business entertaining, when the deal is at risk if you can't share a bottle of wine; at a wedding when you might look churlish if you didn't toast the bride and groom with the requisite glass of champagne; at the zoo when an icecream with the family is only right; or just a quiet G & T to relax you after the legendary hard day at the office.

We're all a bunch of children at heart — have you ever noticed people's faces when the sweet trolley is rolled round? — so why not save your treats for the weekend. Not only is it pleasant to look forward to — a just reward — but the weekends present the greatest temptation, being unstructured, undisciplined and, in a lot of cases, uncontrolled.

The list of bonuses is short, sweet and limited to *five weekly* — in total — in any combination.

1 bonus serving = 3 fl. oz (85 ml) wine — red, white, rosé, champagne, or sherry (the white wine could go further if diluted with soda or Perrier for a spritzer)

or

1 ½ fl. oz (45 ml) spirits (always use slim-line mixers)

or

½ pint (285 ml) beer, lager or cider

or

2 oz (60 g) (normal sized scoop) any icecream

or

2 extra carbohydrate servings

or

2 extra fruit servings

or

2 extra protein servings (excluding the previously banned soft, semi-soft and hard cheese, and eggs, both of which must be eaten in limited quantities as already defined)

That's it! Put another way, you could have one of the following combined bonuses in one week over and above your requisite weekly programme:

> 15 fl. oz (426 ml) champagne (5 × 3 fl. oz/85 ml wine)
> or
> 7½ fl. oz (225 ml) spirits (5 × 1½ fl. oz/45 ml spirits)
> or
> 10 oranges (5 × 2 extra servings fruit)
> or
> 10 oz (285 g) steak (5 × 2 extra servings protein)
> or
> 6 oz (170 g) chocolate icecream and 1 pint (570 ml) lager
> (3 × 2 oz/60 g icecream + 2 × ½ pint/285 ml lager)
> or
> 2 pints (1.1 litres) beer and 3 fl. oz (85 ml) champagne
> (4 × ½ pint /285 ml beer + 1 × 3 fl. oz/85 ml wine)
> or
> 6 oz (170 g) smoked salmon and 6 fl. oz (170 ml) wine
> (3 × 2 extra servings protein + 2 × 3 fl. oz/85 ml wine)
> or
> 10 oz (285 g) granary bread (5 × 2 extra servings carbohydrate)
> or
> 6 oz (170 g) cereal and 4 peaches (3 × 2 extra servings carbohydrate + 2 × 2 extra servings fruit)

These are 'ors' not 'ands', and any combination is OK. In the fortnight's menus following, I've slipped in five bonuses throughout each week — but obviously these are only suggestions. Fill each bonus as you enjoy it in your charts — but don't exceed five during a *week*.

Treat the bonuses as something special, and use them when necessary. Keep on charting your weight and measurements — you 'ain't finished yet! Don't worry, and don't feel guilt-ridden. You'll still lose weight and keep that marvellous feeling of moral superiority.

WEIGHT LOSS ON THE BONUS PROGRAMME

This will naturally not be as great as the first two weeks on the basic programme.

From now on, until you reach your target weight, you'll be losing between 1 ½ and 2 ½ lb (675 g-1.1 kg) per week – sometimes less, and rarely more. Medical and nutritional authorities confirm that a weekly weight loss of 1-2 lb (450-900 g) is advisable while on a sensible diet. Don't get impatient and expect anything miraculous. You're on a programme that's not only life-enhancing, but life-extending.

So you must accept that this is a *permanent* change in your lifestyle. You don't get an educational degree in four weeks, and self-education is what it's all about. Too great a weight loss in too short a time is dangerous physiologically and emotionally. It's counter-productive and you just revert to square one – the weight comes on again and you're no better off, especially in the cheque book.

You can always recognise the man who's just completed his starvation diet or 10-day miracle cure. He's the one in the corner looking like the star of *The Return of the Living Dead*, and probably wolfing down pastries and chocolate gâteaux like there's no tomorrow. Whatever weight he's lost in the last fortnight will go on again in a few days, plus a bit extra for good measure. And he's back where he started, still clueless about his own body and ready to snap up the latest dietary fad.

Keep up your good work. Eat everything and gratefully accept the compliments that you're now beginning to hear.

BONUS PROGRAMME MENUS

Throughout the two weeks ahead, stick to the day's food, and eat it *all* in the 24-hour period. As before, measure your milk and yoghurt allowance carefully. The + after the day heading means that you're now – after the first two weeks – eligible for the wider range of foods and bonuses.

SOME WORDS OF ENCOURAGEMENT

I believe that dieters need encouragement and advice from people who have gone through the same experiences – and have succeeded. I have collected quite a few quotes from businessmen on the subject of alcohol, and you'll find that they include some useful tips.

Here, to start, are some excellent suggestions from a previously overweight senior financial executive in the City of London:

'Non-alcoholic drinks are OK – if you don't want the "influence" effect of alcohol – which most of us don't want most of the time. Long alcoholic drinks are no tastier than non-alcoholic equivalents. I now take an alcoholic drink if I really want one – normally wine at dinner or, occasionally, a whisky. But for all other occasions, I positively prefer the taste and lack of effect of non-alcoholic drinks. Now I drink enthusiastically in order of normal preference:

1. *Ginger beer with lime*
2. *Ginger beer*
3. *Orange and soda*
4. *Grapefruit and tonic*
5. *Perrier or equivalent*
6. *Grape juice*
7. *Lemonade and lime*
8. *Coca-Cola*
9. *Tomato juice*
10. *Apple juice*

I was drinking 2–2½ bottles of wine, or the equivalent, a day in dribs and drabs – lunch, airport, flight, dinner, cocktail party, farewell do, golf club, nightcap, local.'

T.H., Chief Financial Officer

WEEKDAY 1 +

Breakfast

4 fl. oz (115 ml) unsweetened orange juice
1 oz (30 g) wheat flakes, with 1 sliced medium banana,
 and skimmed milk or yoghurt if desired
Tea or coffee unlimited − no sugar

Lunch

3 oz (85 g) smoked salmon
1 oz (30 g) granary bread, with 1 level teaspoon low-fat
 spread
Mixed green salad, with 1 level teaspoon dressing of
 choice
4 oz (115 g) fresh fruit salad, with yoghurt if desired
Tea, coffee, diet drink or mineral water

Dinner

4 oz (115 g) cooked, skinless chicken
Spinach, peas, carrots, with 1 teaspoon low-fat spread
5 oz (140 g) strawberries, with yoghurt if desired
3 fl. oz (85 ml) white wine (*At last*! Make it go twice as
 far by adding Perrier for a spritzer)
Coffee or lemon tea

Bonus = white wine

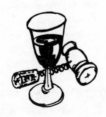

WEEKDAY 2 +

Breakfast

4 fl. oz (115 ml) unsweetened pineapple juice
3 oz (85 g) curd cheese, grilled on 1 oz (30 g) granary
bread (sprinkle with paprika if you like)
Plus as many grilled tomatoes and mushrooms as you
   can eat
Tea, or coffee unlimited – no sugar

Lunch

Artichoke, with 1 level teaspoon low-fat spread, melted,
   or vinaigrette
3 oz (85 g) cooked, skinless turkey
Turnips, green beans, broccoli
5 oz (140 g) strawberries, with yoghurt if desired
Tea, coffee, mineral water or diet drink

Dinner

1 pink grapefruit
3 oz (85 g) grilled Dover sole
Peas, carrots, runner beans, courgettes
3 oz (85 g) cooked potato
Use 2 level teaspoons fat-free spread over all vegetables
4 oz (115 g) fresh fruit salad, with yoghurt if desired
Coffee, lemon tea or mineral water

'I drink Perrier or Diet Coke and pretend.'
Ricci Burns, Founder Ricci Burns

WEEKDAY 3 +

Breakfast

4 oz (115 g) melon
1 oz (30 g) Bran Buds, with 1 oz (30 g) raisins, and
   skimmed milk or yoghurt
Tea or coffee unlimited – no sugar

Lunch

3 oz (85 g) seafood
3 oz (85 g) boiled potato
Asparagus
4 oz (115 g) fresh fruit salad
Coffee, tea, diet drink or mineral water

Dinner

4 oz (115 g) calf's liver
Peas, carrots, parsnips, with 3 level teaspoons low-fat
   spread
1 peach, plus a 2 oz (60 g) scoop vanilla icecream
Coffee, tea or mineral water

Bonus = icecream

'Much as I love it, drink is fattening, lowers the barriers and stimulates the appetite. It also make me tired, which makes me hungry. It is, furthermore, expensive. By cutting down I can afford delicious, non-fattening food treats.'
                                        Eden Phillips, Journalist

WEEKDAY 4 +

Breakfast

1 oz (30 g) Rice Krispies, with 1 sliced medium peach,
and skimmed milk or yoghurt
Tea or coffee unlimited — no sugar

Lunch

3 oz (85 g) lean roast beef
3 oz (85 g) cooked potato
Parsnips, carrots, Brussels sprouts, cauliflower
4 oz (115 g) fresh fruit salad, with yoghurt if desired
Coffee, lemon tea, mineral water or diet drink

Dinner

4 oz (115 g) melon
4 oz (115 g) lemon sole
Mixed green salad, with 3 level teaspoons vinaigrette,
salad cream or mayonnaise
1 kiwi fruit
Coffee, tea or mineral water

*'I drink little alcohol, but large amounts of water, both
natural and mineral, lots of fruit juice and lots of Diet
Coke, ginger ale and lemonade.'*
Andy Cappucinni, Vice-President, Head of Trading,
Smith Barney, Investment Bankers

WEEKDAY 5+

Breakfast

4 fl. oz (115 ml) unsweetened apple juice
1 oz (30 g) Bran Flakes, with 1 sliced or chopped apple,
  and yoghurt or skimmed milk
Tea or coffee unlimited − no sugar

Lunch

3 oz (85 g) plainly cooked game (pheasant, quail,
  pigeon, rabbit, venison − still no extras!)
Mushrooms, green beans, peas, with 1 level teaspoon
  low-fat spread
5 oz (140 g) raspberries, with yoghurt if desired
Coffee, tea or mineral water

Dinner

4 oz (115 g) fresh fruit salad
4 oz (115 g) smoked salmon
1 oz (30 g) granary bread, with 2 level teaspoons low-fat
  spread
6 oz (170 g) grapes
Coffee, tea or mineral water

Bonus = 2 extra fruit servings

'I drink a good deal of water − we all are mostly water, and we're losing it all the time. Eventually we'll end up like dried-up prunes!'
David Quilter, Actor and Dedicated Jogger

WEEKEND 1 +

Breakfast

2 tangerines, in sections
1 oz (30 g) Cornflakes, with skimmed milk or yoghurt
Tea or coffee unlimited — no sugar

Lunch

3 oz (85 g) chicken *tikka* at your favourite Indian
  restaurant
3 oz (85 g) rice, and all the vegetables you can handle,
  plus a *raitha* (cucumber or mint in natural yoghurt), the
  perfect partner for the chicken. (You're not allowed
  any fat today, because the vegetables are bound to be
  in a sauce containing a proportion of fat.)
½ pint (285 ml) beer
Tea, coffee or mineral water

Dinner

4 oz (115 g) melon
4 oz (115 g) lean roast beef
Parsnips, carrots, peas, cauliflower
8 oz (225 g) fresh fruit salad
Coffee

Bonus = beer

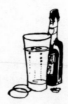

WEEKEND 2 +

Brunch

4 oz (115 g) melon
2-egg omelette, made with 1 level teaspoon low-fat
   spread
Plus 1 oz (30 g) grated Cheddar cheese, and as many
   grilled tomatoes and mushrooms as you want
1 oz (30 g) granary roll, with 1 level teaspoon low-fat
   spread
Tea or coffee unlimited — no sugar

Dinner

1 pink grapefruit
4 oz (115 g) roast veal
Broccoli, green peas, carrots, runner beans, with 1 level
   teaspoon low-fat spread
3 oz (85 g) cooked potatoes
8 oz (225 g) fresh fruit salad, with yoghurt if desired
3 fl. oz (85 ml) red wine
Coffee

Bonus = red wine

*'While I love wine, I will "sit" on a full glass for lengthy
periods to restrict the intake.'*
               Graham White, Television Executive, Australia

WEEKDAY 6 +

Breakfast

1 oz (30 g) Cornflakes, with 1 medium sliced banana,
  and yoghurt or skimmed milk
Tea or coffee unlimited — no sugar

Lunch

3 oz (85 g) fresh poached or grilled salmon
3 oz (85 g) cooked potato
Peas, carrots
5 oz (140 g) raspberries, with yoghurt if desired
Coffee, tea, diet drink or mineral water

Dinner

4 oz (115 g) cooked, skinless chicken
Parsnips, green beans, cauliflower, with 3 level
  teaspoons low-fat spread
2 peaches
Coffee, diet drink or mineral water

*'Mineral water with lime or Diet Coke covers most of my
needs. "I'm driving", or "I've got to take the baby-sitter
home" is another nice one-liner to show a responsible
adult, or "I'm a Muslim". It confuses people enough to
allow a soft drink to be ordered.'*
Tony Aplin, Chairman, APA

WEEKDAY 7+

Breakfast

4 fl. oz (115 ml) unsweetened pineapple juice
2 poached eggs, on 2 oz (60 g) granary toast
Plus as many grilled tomatoes and mushrooms as you
    want
Coffee or tea unlimited — no sugar

Lunch

4 oz (115 g) lean roast lamb
Green beans, carrots, broccoli
8 oz (225 g) fresh fruit salad, with yoghurt if desired
Coffee, lemon tea or mineral water

Dinner

Asparagus, with 1 level teaspoon low-fat spread
3 oz (85 g) tuna, with an enormous salad, and 2 level
    teaspoons dressing of choice
1 peach
Coffee, lemon tea or mineral water

Bonus = 2 extra servings protein

'Heredity, an attentive partner, good luck and constant
vigilance help your diet. Cut down on alcohol and desserts,
and include exercise daily.'

Alan Bacon, Partner, Tootsies Restaurants

WEEKDAY 8 +

Breakfast

1 oz (30 g) Bran Buds, with 1 oz (30 g) raisins, and
skimmed milk or yoghurt
Tea or coffee unlimited — no sugar

Lunch

3 oz (85 g) grilled Dover sole
Large mixed green salad, with 1 level teaspoon
vinaigrette
1 kiwi fruit
Diet drink, mineral water or lemon tea

Dinner

1 grapefruit
Cottage pie (4 oz/115 g meat sauce, topped with
3 oz/85 g mashed potato, augmented if you like with
mashed cauliflower, see page 40)
Peas, carrots, parsnips, with 2 level teaspoons low-fat
spread
1 peach
Coffee, or mineral water

WEEKDAY 9 +

Breakfast

4 fl. oz (115 ml) unsweetened orange juice
1 oz (30 g) porridge cooked slowly in skimmed milk (see
   page 36), with 1 sliced banana (add during cooking,
   it's fabulous)
Coffee or tea unlimited − no sugar

Lunch

4 oz (115 g) melon
3 oz (85 g) prawn, lobster or crab salad, with 1 level
   teaspoon dressing of choice
6 oz (170 g) baked potato (with yoghurt, onion and
   chives perhaps)
Coffee, tea, diet drink or mineral water

Dinner

3 oz (85 g) cooked, skinless turkey
Brussels sprouts, peas, carrots, runner beans, with 2
   level teaspoons low-fat spread
3 oz (85 g) grapes
1 oz (30 g) hard cheese plus 1 oz (30 g) wholewheat
   rolls
Coffee, tea or mineral water

Bonus = 2 extra carbohydrate servings

WEEKDAY 10+

Breakfast

1 oz (30 g) Bran Flakes, with 1 sliced medium peach,
   and yoghurt or skimmed milk
Coffee or tea unlimited — no sugar

Lunch

3 oz (85 g) smoked salmon
2 oz (60 g) granary bread, with 2 level teaspoons low-fat
   spread
5 oz (140 g) raspberries, with yoghurt if desired
Coffee, lemon tea or mineral water

Dinner

1 grapefruit
4 oz (115 g) cooked, skinless chicken
3 oz (85 g) wholemeal pasta
Carrots, green beans, asparagus, with 1 level teaspoon
   low-fat spread
1 kiwi fruit
Coffee or mineral water

Bonus = 2 extra carbohydrate servings

WEEKEND 3+

Breakfast

2 tangerines, in sections
2-egg omelette, made with 1 level teaspoon low-fat
spread
1 oz (30 g) granary toast
Coffee or tea unlimited — no sugar

Lunch

3 oz (85 g) curd cheese
Enormous mixed salad, with 1 level teaspoon dressing
1 peach
Coffee, tea or diet drink

Dinner

4 oz (115 g) melon
4 oz (115 g) grilled fillet steak
3 oz (85 g) cooked potato
Peas, carrots, sprouts, parsnips, with 1 level teaspoon
low-fat spread
4 oz (115 g) fresh fruit salad, with yoghurt if desired
3 fl. oz (85 ml) red wine
Coffee

Bonus = red wine

*'I suppose part of me (I'm not sure which part) wishes I
could give up drink completely, since the nutritive value is
so small, but then the loss of the other less-easily measured
values might out-weigh the benefits of giving up.'*
Pete Atkin, Producer, BBC

WEEKEND 4 +

Eat a couple of apples — or another two fruit servings —
throughout the day whenever you like.

Brunch

5 oz (140 g) raspberries, with yoghurt
2 scrambled eggs, made with 1 level teaspoon low-fat
  spread
Plus 1 oz (30 g) grated Cheddar cheese and as many
  grilled tomatoes and mushrooms as you want
1 oz (30 g) wholewheat roll, with 1 level teaspoon low-
  fat spread
Coffee or tea unlimited — no sugar

Dinner

4 oz (115 g) melon
4 oz (115 g) plainly cooked pork (*no* crackling)
Peas, carrots, broccoli, green beans, with 1 level
  teaspoon low-fat spread
3 oz (85 g) cooked rice
3 fl. oz (85 ml) white wine or ½ pint (285 ml) cider
Coffee, mineral water or diet drink

Bonus = white wine or cider

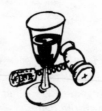

SPECIAL DAY

(out for dinner with your partner and using up 4 bonuses)

Breakfast

2 satsumas in sections
1 oz (30 g) Bran Flakes, with skimmed milk or yoghurt
Coffee or tea unlimited — no sugar

Lunch

3 oz (85 g) curd cheese
Enormous mixed salad, with 1 level teaspoon dressing
5 oz (140 g) strawberries with yoghurt, if desired
Coffee, tea or mineral water

Dinner

6 fl. oz (170 ml) vegetable soup
6 oz (170 g) grilled fillet steak
6 oz (170 g) new potatoes
Peas, carrots, runner beans with 2 level teaspoons low-
   fat spread
2 oz (60 g) icecream, plus
4 oz (115 g) fresh fruit salad (non liqueur-based variety)
3 fl. oz (85 ml) red wine
1 ½ fl. oz (45 ml) cognac
Coffee
(No after dinner mints!)

Bonuses = wine, cognac, carbohydrate, icecream

BONUS PROGRAMME FOOD DIARY

1st Week

Total number of weekly bonuses. Do not exceed five. ☐☐☐☐☐

Day	Morning	Afternoon	Evening	Servings Allowance
1				4 fruits ☐☐☐☐ 3 fats ☐☐☐ milk/yoghurt ☐ 7 protein ☐☐☐☐ ☐☐☐ 2 carbohydrates ☐☐ Bonus . . . . ☐
2				4 fruits ☐☐☐☐ 3 fats ☐☐☐ milk/yoghurt ☐ 7 protein ☐☐☐☐ ☐☐☐ 2 carbohydrates ☐☐ Bonus . . . . ☐
3				4 fruits ☐☐☐☐ 3 fats ☐☐☐ milk/yoghurt ☐ 7 protein ☐☐☐☐ ☐☐☐ 2 carbohydrates ☐☐ Bonus . . . . ☐

4	4 fruits 3 fats milk/yoghurt 7 protein 2 carbohydrates Bonus		
5	4 fruits 3 fats milk/yoghurt 7 protein 2 carbohydrates Bonus		
6	4 fruits 3 fats milk/yoghurt 7 protein 2 carbohydrates Bonus		
7	4 fruits 3 fats milk/yoghurt 7 protein 2 carbohydrates Bonus		

Weight after Week One on Bonus Programme . . . .

BONUS PROGRAMME FOOD DIARY

2nd Week

Total number of weekly bonuses. **Do not exceed five.** ☐☐☐☐☐

Day	Morning	Afternoon	Evening	Servings Allowance
8				4 fruits ☐☐☐☐ 3 fats ☐☐☐ milk/yoghurt ☐ ☐☐☐ 7 protein ☐☐☐☐ 2 carbohydrates ☐☐ Bonus . . . . ☐
9				4 fruits ☐☐☐☐ 3 fats ☐☐☐ milk/yoghurt ☐ ☐☐☐ 7 protein ☐☐☐☐ 2 carbohydrates ☐☐ Bonus . . . . ☐
10				4 fruits ☐☐☐☐ 3 fats ☐☐☐ milk/yoghurt ☐ ☐☐☐ 7 protein ☐☐☐☐ 2 carbohydrates ☐☐ Bonus . . . . ☐

11				4 fruits ☐☐☐☐ 3 fats ☐☐☐ milk/yoghurt ☐☐ ☐ 7 protein ☐☐☐☐ ☐☐☐ 2 carbohydrates ☐☐ Bonus .... ☐
12				4 fruits ☐☐☐☐ 3 fats ☐☐☐ milk/yoghurt ☐☐ ☐ 7 protein ☐☐☐☐ ☐☐☐ 2 carbohydrates ☐☐ Bonus .... ☐
13				4 fruits ☐☐☐☐ 3 fats ☐☐☐ milk/yoghurt ☐☐ ☐ 7 protein ☐☐☐☐ ☐☐☐ 2 carbohydrates ☐☐ Bonus .... ☐
14				4 fruits ☐☐☐☐ 3 fats ☐☐☐ milk/yoghurt ☐☐ ☐ 7 protein ☐☐☐☐ ☐☐☐ 2 carbohydrates ☐☐ Bonus .... ☐

Weight after Week Two on Bonus Programme ....

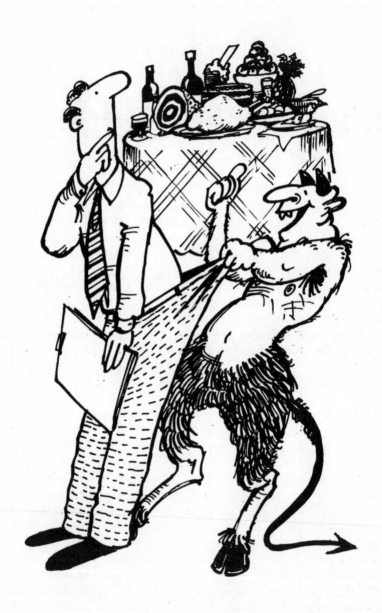

CHAPTER FIVE

The Temptations, or 'Oh Come On, Harry, Just This Once . . .'

You've accomplished miracles in the last four weeks: the first two you really persevered and lost x pounds; in the second two, you allowed yourself a few bonuses – the odd glass of wine or spirits, a little rice or boiled potato – and you *still* continued to lose weight. So here you are, feeling and looking much better. The danger now is not of losing heart but of giving way to what might seem like justifiable temptation, to one of your favourite pre-diet foods – chocolate or biscuits, say – or to more alcohol than is allowed on the programme. But *pause* – before you fall, and think carefully. Getting to know thyself will point the way to control.

BINGES

Before having even *one taste* of a favourite forbidden food, stop! For there's no such thing as eating only one chocolate from the box. First you eat one, then the top layer, then the bottom layer, and then you'll throw the box away to destroy the evidence. There's no such thing as 'one thin slice' of gâteau. The first slice is exactly that – the first of many. There's no such thing as only one biscuit from the package. You'll eat the lot, like the biscuit freak who, realising his particular addiction, swore that he'd only eat the broken biscuits from the package. And, amazingly enough, he always managed to drop the package on his way home ...

Don't beat about the bush, you know basically where the trouble lies. You know *your* binge foods: it's chocolate, it's peanuts or crisps, or it's boiled sweets. All of them absolute *no-nos.*

Or it might be cheese. 'Nothing wrong with cheese, is there? Good, solid, dairy food – good for you!' Sure, it's good for you, but it's no good for you in the *quantities* you're eating. For cheese is very high on the caution list (yet another glance at the fat content chart on page 39 will explain precisely why). It's always there, at the back of the fridge, ready to be eaten. Often before you've even taken off your coat, you might have a big hunk of cheese, a healthy wedge of French bread, and a generous spreading of butter. 'Can't be any harm in that – all good healthy foods.'

Yes, they are, but only in the right quantities, and at the correct weights. It's so easy to cut a wedge of cheese weighing a quarter of a pound and wolf it down right there and then, with your back to the door as if anticipating the imminent dropping of a nuclear missile.

This is the road to disaster. You must put the same amount of planning into your food and drink as you do into other aspects of your life. You don't buy a word-processor because the colour is attractive. You don't employ a marketing manager because your neighbour's brother-in-law went to school with him. You consider, you judge, you decide. You follow a considered plan. And that's what you have to do with your eating programme. Follow a considered plan of action.

Always be conscious of food weights. A 1 oz (30 g) block of cheese (what you're allowed on the bonus programme as part of your protein allowance) doesn't seem a great deal – but when it's grated it's a substantial amount. And grated, it has the bonus of taking longer to eat. Following the rule that we all eat far too quickly, I've often caused great hilarity by eating cereal and soup with a teaspoon. But there's method in my apparent madness, as I've said before: the result is far more satisfying for the mind and stomach.

Audrey Eyton, of *F-Plan* fame, stated that you eat what you buy. So true. If you don't buy it, you won't be tempted. 'What the eye doesn't see', etc. Food shopping is a huge problem, but whether it's a single or shared responsibility, or a chore handled solely by your partner, it can only be solved by foresight, and that word again − planning. If *you* know what your binge foods are, it's more than likely that your partner knows them as well; cooperation is vital if you are not to fall off your lighter-weight perch.

But what if you do binge? In all probability, that occasion will arise. Perhaps a similar situation to this:

Saturday night has been a disaster − food and drink-wise, that is. Too much rich sauce over the fillet steak, too many profiteroles, the wine, the brandy, and everybody telling you: 'Just this once, Harry, forget about your wretched diet.' Most of us react to over-indulgence of this sort in one of two ways . . . both equally ineffective.

Reaction A

'My God, I've really blown it now . . . what an idiot. I just don't have the self-control or discipline. To hell with it anyway . . . I'll start again next month, and I'll be 100 per cent angelic. I'll cheer myself up and have a big fry-up for breakfast, bacon, fried bread, the lot.'

Result

A gloomy sense of 'failed-again' guilt, and a great loss of self-image and confidence.

Reaction B

'I've really made an ass of myself this time . . . but, by God, I'm going to make up for it. Only black coffee and yoghurt today. I'll even it out, starvation never hurt anybody.'

Result

Headaches, edginess, lethargy, and an inability to deal with life, plus irritability with those around you.

OK, so what is the magic answer: There ain't one – magical, that is! But to inflict the minimal damage to yourself, adopt a pragmatic approach. Right. You were an idiot, you did go berserk. But that was yesterday. Don't live that binge over and over again. Stop the self-flagellation and forget it.

Today's a new day, and you're starting from scratch. And that means eating everything you have to – not skipping any of your required foods, and not cutting down on serving sizes or the amount of servings. Don't ever starve yourself to lose weight or make up for a binge. And don't put yourself down with thoughts of how awful you are. You're human, and face complex factors that have to be dealt with on a day-to-day basis. The binge happened yesterday, and you'll try not to repeat the mistake. You knew well in advance about the dinner party; next time you'll go better prepared. Like everything else, the better the planning, the more successful the outcome.

But a tolerant attitude about yourself does work. Not a permissive attitude, mind you, never that. But a tolerance towards your own foibles and crises. Just eat well and plentifully every day. Enjoy your food, take time to eat it, and be prepared for those temptation items.

The crisis has passed and you've handled it well or not so well. But it has passed. Just get on with living with yourself – and everyone else – content in mind and body.

I'm beginning to sound like a latter-day evangelist again, so here endeth the California pyscho-babble ... but not before a touch of fantasy. Of course, we all fantasise ... we all escape to Nirvana ... the amazing magic pill. Take before bed, and lo and behold, you wake up with the body of Sylvester Stallone. A trifle less muscled, perhaps a shade more intellectual, but the body is fine.

Alas, the magic pill is an illusion. (And a good thing too. A community solely populated by Sylvester Stallones and Bo Dereks is just too much.) In the cold, grey dawn of reality, that's *you* glumly staring back at yourself in the full-length mirror after your shower. But *tomorrow*, or perhaps two months from tomorrow, that body could be transformed into a leaner, healthier, more energetic you ... alert and confident, and in

CONTROL. Perhaps not Sylvester (who needs all those biceps anyway), but a man with a secure self-image and that wonderful sense of well-being that comes from a healthy, intelligent eating programme.

CHOCOHOLISM

What's the most common problem facing businessmen on a diet? No, it isn't drink — it's actually chocolate and other sweet things.

The Scene: The local newsagent's shop

The Time: The present — 8.30 am

The Cast: Newsagent's assistant
                  Assorted customers, mainly male
                  Me

Scenario: I am patiently waiting for the assistant to dig out a copy of *The Economist* (for I do have a life beyond weight control). Assorted customers enter, are served and leave. Four purchase cigarettes, seven collect newspapers but, with the exception of one spartan soul, all buy chocolate.

Total Running Time: 3 minutes

Total Quantity of
Chocolate
Purchased: 14 bars

Incredible. And then, to cap it all, in *The Times* shortly afterwards the proud boast: 'Britain consumes more sweets and chocolate than any other European country. Confectionery sales in the UK exceeded 2.5 billion last year [1986].'

Musing on these events in my rare moments of meditation, I

recalled the charming Harry, prince of chocoholics. A tall, tanned daily jogger, weekly squash and tennis player, and father of two, he was nearly obsessive in his observance of his food programme. But with that one fatal weakness. You guessed it — chocolate! Disaster generally struck Harry while doing his duty as sales director for a computer company, often travelling, and always with a very tough schedule.

He would creep furtively into the class so late that I was forced to weigh him when the remaining group had departed. He'd then confess in hushed tones that he had again succumbed to temptation and fallen into the chocolate pleasures of the flesh.

One evening Harry made his classic entrance looking so shame-faced that I couldn't resist the chance to preach a sermonette, with poor Harry as the supplicant. It appeared that he'd just departed from the motorway sweet shop, where he'd consumed a few bon-bons . . . quite a few!

'How many is a few, Harry?'

'Oh, just a few . . . a couple of Curly-Wurlys, three Kit-Kats, an Aero Bar, two Mars Bars, and something made of coconut . . . '

A hushed silence from the group.

And through the stillness came the voice of the Reverend Michael, his tones of accusation cutting to the very heart of the trembling transgressor. 'You'll surely pay for that binge, Harry. I trust you feel sick as a dog.'

And came the muted reply of the sinner: 'No, I don't actually . . . in fact, I could eat another six!'

Uproar and rapid deflation of the guru.

The confectionery industry and, in particular, their ingenious advertising and marketing agencies have a great deal to answer for. The figures for obesity, heart disease and dental decay prove the point. Try to forget 'A choccy a day helps you work, rest and play'. A healthier version runs: 'A choccy a day makes your teeth rot away.'

'But, oh!' you cry, with an injured tone. 'They're just great when you're feeling tired, and everybody knows they're instant energy.'

Rubbish. You get as much instant energy from oranges, grapes, plums, satsumas and raisins. And fruit is just as easily available and portable as a chocolate bar. Don't take my word for it ... speak to any professional sports coach.

And while you're at it, take a look at this analysis of a mini Swiss Roll and its ingredients: 'Black cherry flavour filling (Sugar, gelling agent E440A, Citric Acid, Acidity Regulator E330, Flavouring, Colours E122, E132, Wheat Flour, Sugar, Starch, Whole Egg, Butter, Invert Sugar Syrup, Marshmallow, Glucose Syrup, Albumen, Emulsifiers E470, E471, Skimmed Milk Powder, Animal & Vegetable Fats, Glycerine, Salt, Colours E120, E110, E202, Preservative.' (Geoffrey Cannon in a review of *E for Additives* by Maurice Hanssen, Thorsons.)

Worrying reading? You bet it is.

And don't be fooled by the 'new' health bars containing no sugar. In a lot of cases, they've simply substituted honey or glucose for the sugar. And while I'm loathe to contradict Barbara Cartland, honey is as fattening and tooth-rotting as sugar, as is any ingredient ending in 'OSE' (glucose, dextrose, etc.).

Heaven knows, it's hard to resist. On every side, you're bombarded with scenes of nubile beauties simulating oral sex with a chocolate bar on a Polynesian island, teams of macho lorry drivers munching away while doing their trans-continental bit for Britain, superpower meetings brought to a successful conclusion by the production of a particular chocolate. Don't be a chump ... don't fall for it.

You've been successful in your career. Every day you make intelligent, thoughtful decisions. Separating the hype from the facts is an integral part of your life. Take a long, hard look at the pros and cons.

First the 'cons'. Chocolate and sweets

★ damage your health

★ ruin your teeth

★ make you fat and *keep* you fat

★ are addictive — the more you eat, the more you want

★ cost a lot of money — and that's not the only cost.

HOW MUCH SUGAR IN THE FOOD YOU EAT?

1 average teaspoon = 5 g sugar. The starred foods (*) are also high in fat.

Food	Amount	No of Teaspoons of Sugar
Confectionery		
Toffees, boiled sweets*	1	1
Kit-Kat	1x2-finger bar	3
Maltesers	1 standard packet	4½
Creme Egg (41 g)	1	5
Crunchie	1 bar	5
Polo Mints	1 tube	6
Chocolate*	1 × 2oz (60g) bar	7
Dolly Mixtures	1 small box	20½
Cakes		
Scone	1	½
Currant bun	1	1
Fruit pie	1 individual	2
Jam tart	1 individual	3
Iced sponge cake	1 medium slice	5
Biscuits		
Digestive*	1	½
Plain (Marie, Rich Tea)	1	1
Ginger Nut	1	1
Chocolate digestive*	1	2
Rich Sweet (Custard Creme)	1	2
Drinks		
Tonic Water	1 medium bottle	2
Drinking chocolate	3 teaspoons	2

Drinks (continued)

Lemonade	1 glass	2½
Orange/Lemon squash	1 glass	2½
Vimto	1 glass	3
Lucozade	1 glass	3½
Ginger ale	1 medium bottle	4
Bitter lemon	1 medium bottle	5
Blackcurrant cordial (diluted)	1x7 fl. oz (200 ml) glass	6
Cola	1 can (330 ml)	7

Desserts

Icecream*	1 scoop	2
Instant custard	1 portion	2
Canned rice pudding	1 bowl	2½
Fruit yoghurt	5 oz (140 g) carton	3
Choc ice*	1	3
Sponge pudding with jam/syrup*	1 medium slice	5½
Jelly	⅓ packet made up	5
Canned fruit in syrup	1 bowl	5
Instant Whip	¼ packet made up	10

Breakfast Cereals

Shredded Wheat	1 biscuit	0
Porridge Oats	1 oz (30 g)	0
Weetabix	1 biscuit	¼
Sugar Puffs	1 bowl	3

Sweet Spreads

Honey	2 teaspoons	2
Jam	2 teaspoons	2
Marmalade	2 teaspoons	2

Then the 'pros'. Chocolate and sweets

★ provide instant energy (as previously stated, nonsense)

★ are easily available and portable (so are oranges, plums and raisins)

★ are delicious – granted, but you can't win 'em all, as they say.

Harry, the Prince of Chocoholics, is not an isolated addict – for addiction it certainly is. Chocolate contains a drug, caffeine, the same drug that is present in coffee, strong tea, cocoa and Coca-Cola. Chocoholics make up the largest section of binge eaters in any weight-control group. That's right, even greater than the section addicted to the demon drink.

Chocolates also contain an amine called tyramine, which has fairly recently been isolated as one of the major causes of migraine headaches. London's Migraine Centre confirms what many sufferers already know to their cost, that chocolate plays an unfortunately large part in their affliction. And I can personally vouch for the authenticity of this. On a recent trip to Normandy I was so taken with the French custom of a large bowl of hot chocolate in the morning that I introduced it to our château in Chiswick. It took only three days' quaffing before I was in bed with blinding headaches that I'd never experienced previously. A call to the doctor established that the cause was the chocolate. I stopped and so did the headaches. I'll never forget the misery and the pain of those migraines, and have every sympathy with those who suffer from them.

Just to add the icing to the cake, if I may (and that's an unfortunate turn of phrase in the circumstances), take another look at the sugar content of everyday confectionery items on pages 110-111. As well as posing potential health hazards such as migraine (and also being associated with allergies), chocolate is plain *fattening*. I could go on *ad nauseam*, but I hope I've already awakened you to the terrors that lurk therein . . .

THE DEMON DRINK

Chocolate and sweets may well be the most common problem for dieting businessmen, but Public Enemy Number Two is unquestionably the overwhelming pervasiveness of drinking in every aspect of our society: the glass or glasses of wine at lunch, the beer after the office, the welcoming G & T on arrival at home, the half-bottle of wine with dinner, the brandy afterwards, the celebratory champagne on special occasions (or occasions you convince yourself are celebratory)!

I'm not advocating total abstinence. Certainly, many recent studies have reported that drink in moderation can be an aid to a healthy life, and that moderate drinkers are no less fit than their teetotal colleagues. But the common word in all the surveys and reports is *moderation*. And that doesn't mean cutting down from two bottles of wine daily to one and a half bottles. It *means* moderation.

If you've followed the basic programme, you will have given up wine and spirits for the first two weeks. You may have done it without enthusiasm perhaps, but nevertheless you will have done it. If you are now on the bonus programme, you are allowed bonuses in the quantities listed in Chapter 4. Just to remind you:

3 fl. oz (85 ml) any wine — white, red, rosé, champagne or sherry
1 ½ fl. oz (45 ml) — any spirits
½ pint (285 ml) — any beer, lager or cider

Any one of those quantities can be enjoyed, if desired, five times a week. Therefore if you're using all your bonuses in drink only, your weekly quota works out at:

15 fl. oz (425 ml) wine
or
7 ½ fl. oz (225ml) spirits
or
2 ½ pints (1.4 litres) beer, lager or cider
or
Any combination totalling five bonuses.

Do I hear a concerted chorus of groans? Surely not! Aren't you proud, having disciplined yourself to give up alcohol completely for a fortnight? Haven't you gained a distinctive air of moral superiority at the office and at home? Don't you feel just a bit more sharp, energetic and fit? Aren't you sleeping better, feeling better and looking better? Come on now, you know you are.

And in addition you have a lot of factors helping you to keep the faith. We are all aware now of the dangers involved in drinking too much, and the effect it can have on the whole body, let alone the poor liver. No longer does a charge of drunken driving receive a jolly response of: 'Be more careful next time, Harry.' And it appears that even greater and stronger legal methods are in the pipeline. 'Drinking and driving' is a target of understandable moral and social concern.

The diminishing image of the 'macho male' has also played a crucial role. The beer-swilling, falling-down bar fly has been joined by the embarrassing, over-loud, red-faced dinner guest whom everybody takes great care to avoid. What you experience when you're sober and he isn't is a revelation. Doesn't he realise what an idiot he's making of himself? Of course he doesn't. He's just 'one over the eight', or 'feeling more relaxed'. But what he appears to you and the world is sad, pathetic and insecure.

The *need* for booze in a professional and social context is changing too, both here and in the States. In New York virtually no-one drinks now; it's just not fashionable any more, and what happens there seems to reach the rest of us a few years later. It's quite fashionable now to *not* drink, to show that you're caring about your health, your career and your family.

However, you did give up the booze for two weeks, so you're hardly alcoholic. I'm simply trying to make the point that you're kidding yourself if you feel that two weeks of total abstinence is all that's required. It isn't. What you have to decide and act on now is a plan of control, and you must limit your intake for the rest of your life. Yes, for the rest of your life. A somewhat daunting prospect. Planning and control are the answer.

I've been through a few of the basics already, but here are a few more practical and behavioural tips.

Mineral waters aren't confined to Perrier and Pellagrino. Try

Vichy, Ashbourne and dozens of others. They all have their own distinctive tastes; some are fizzy, some still.

Try a diet soft drink – not only Coke, but Diet Pepsi, 7-Up, Tango, Lilt, 1-Cal, Ginger ale and tonic. As I said before, look for the *no sugar* assurance on the label. Beware, too, of the tonics: not all so-called low-calorie tonics are low-calorie enough when you're dieting. Avoid those that say low-calorie and nothing else. Use the brands that spell out the exact calorie count.

Fruit juices are fine as substitutes for alcohol. Make sure they're unsweetened and don't drink them in vast quantities. Any unsweetened fruit juice is part of your daily allowance, but a 4 fl. oz (114 ml) helping is the ration – or you can have two extra servings as one bonus on the bonus programme – so keep a note on your chart.

Combine your mineral water with the permitted wine, red or white. It's very pleasant and refreshing, and makes your wine allowance travel twice the distance.

Try a St Clement's: orange juice, with a lemon slice and some soda.

Try the non-alcoholic wines and beers – there are quite a few on the market now. I'm no expert on wine and beer, far from it. But Paul Levy, Food and Wine Editor of the *Observer*, definitely is. His pre-Christmas 1987 article on wines, beers and a cider that were low in alcohol or alcohol-free was based on drinking and driving: however, low in alcohol also means low in calories, and these drinks are therefore very relevant for The Businessman's Diet. He says:

'British food labelling regulations allow drinks with a maximum alcohol strength of 0.05 per cent ... to call themselves "alcohol free". Many fruit juices and soft drinks contain such traces of alcohol. The regulations say that the hideous word "De-alcoholised" may be used for drinks in the range 0.05 – 0.5 per cent. Most producers have opted for the less technical sounding term, "low alcohol" for bevvies in this strength band, though this term is also acceptable for higher-strength drinks, from 0.5 – 1.2 per cent.

'Though the legal maximum strength for a drink on which duty is not payable is 1.2 per cent, the trade generally works to 1 per cent, in order to avoid problems arising at the borderline. "Light" beers go from 1.6 to 2.5 per cent. It is at this level of alcohol that most people experience physiological effects, and that HM Customs and Excise begin to take an interest in the contents of the can or bottle!'

I list below a few of those he tasted − but did not necessarily recommend! − with their percentage of alcohol per volume:

WINES

	% Alcohol
Eisberg	0.05
Jung	0.05
Masson Light	less than 0.5

BEERS AND LAGERS

	%Alcohol
Clausthaler	0.6
Highway	1
Kaliber	0.05
Warteck	0.5
White Label	1

CIDER

	%Alcohol
Taunton Cool	3

Mr Levy finished off his article with a comment about an alcohol-free wine being served with soda as a spritzer: 'A refreshing and inoffensive way to enjoy a party and be able to drive home with a clear conscience and a clean licence'.

Yes, alcohol can be an enjoyable part of your life. In moderation, that is, to preserve not only your conscience and licence, but your figure and your health. In excess it can destroy your career, your reputation, your family and you.

Here are a few tips.

A highly successful client of mine who runs restaurants and nightclubs always makes an arrangement with the barman when he's entertaining. Whilst his guests receive what they order, he is served only tonic water with a slice of lemon. They assume there is gin or vodka in there too.

And as a guest, it's remarkable how little attention is actually paid to you as long as you have a full glass. The full glass is the key — it doesn't matter to your host or hostess what's in it, nor will it occur to them. It's full and they are, therefore, doing their duty as far as entertaining and hospitality are concerned. Have a glass of water or mineral water alongside your wine, and use this to quench your thirst.

The medicinal white lie is always effective too — a *sotto voce* muttering of, 'Sorry, can't, my doctor, you know ...' works wonders. Although it does leave a vague intimation of your imminent expiry, in the final throes of beri-beri. A worthwhile ploy nonetheless. And the ultimate excuse is one used by a Wall Street trader, who is teetotal from choice, but who feels his refusal of a drink lessens his tough trading image. On entering the room, he counters the traditional question: 'And what would you like to drink?' with a slightly apologetic whisper of: 'Sorry to be a nuisance, but I'm AA.' The concerned host then spends the remainder of the evening trying frantically not to give him any drink at all!

For more alcohol-related advice from other dieters, look back to the suggested menus for the Bonus Diet.

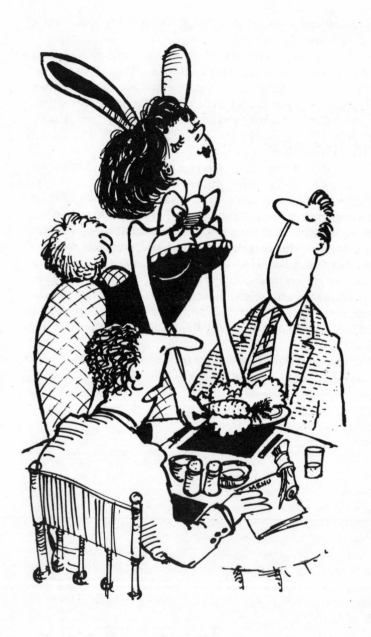

CHAPTER 6

Eating Out, or How to Survive the Business Lunch

Great — you've now made it through untold amounts of sage advice on what to eat, what *not* to eat, when to eat, when *not* to eat, the choices, the quantities, and the temptations. But now we'll move on to the mean streets of commercial practicality. And there's nothing like the business lunch or dinner to bring you back to earth with a thud.

Before we start, let's make a deal. I'll forget lengthy paragraphs of facts and preaching if you'll forego those excuses that you hope will exonerate you from reading on. Let's see, there's ...

'Old Charlie always expects a slap-up lunch at the best place in town',
and

'We always split at least one or two bottles — it's become sort of a tradition',
and

'He'll think we're having liquidity problems — it's the company's way of saying thank-you',
and

'I realise that it sounds pompous, but I must be seen, as a senior executive, to be entertaining a valued client in a generous, hospitable, and proper manner.'

Only the last excuse has merit. Of course, you must be seen to be hospitable, caring and competent. But that doesn't entail staggering back to the office at 4 o'clock, feeling like the living dead, and somewhat hazy as to where you were, with whom, and the original object of the exercise.

ADVANCE PLANNING

The answer for the dieting businessman is to plan ahead, to plan the meal like you do any other project. Judge the situation carefully: are you the guest or the host? In either case, you're the one in charge.

If you're the host, you can pick the time, the place and the menu. After all, you are picking up the bill. If you're the guest, you're the quarry – so flex your muscles and do the same.

'There's a great place on Charlotte Street – Greek.'

'How about roast beef at the Connaught?'

'They do wonderful Dover sole at Wheelers.'

Host or guest, you choose the battlefield and the weapons. And this means that you can choose Greek (char-grilled kebabs and lots of salad); the Connaught for that lean beef with lots of salad; or the sole grilled with a salad, and perhaps a boiled new potato or two.

The choices of where to go are endless, and can fit in with your food preferences. But the quantities and scope of the meal in relation to the rest of your dieting day are highly dependent on pre-planning.

Right. You're off to the Connaught for the infamous slap-up lunch with Charlie. Well and good. But if you've planned breakfast or dinner at home, adjust them accordingly. Use your charts to work out what you can have or can't have, and prepare with a lightish breakfast, to be followed in the evening by a similarly light dinner.

And don't leave this to the last minute. Announcing to your partner on the doorstep at 7.30 pm that 'I took Old Charlie for lunch, darling – so it's one poached egg and black coffee for me, I'm afraid' will not go down well. Especially if your partner has spent a good part of the day preparing a splendid (but dietary) *haute cuisine* dinner. The potential strain on domestic harmony should never be under-estimated.

Business lunches or dinners are rarely organised at the last minute, so if you've arranged one a week before, make sure you plan ahead, and make sure your partner knows all about it. Your partner merits and requires 100 per cent cooperation, and the support you'll receive in return will prove a wonderful investment in your health and your relationships.

Another tip to help you along is to make the appointment early rather than late, and have a cup of coffee or a piece of fruit before you get there. Otherwise, you'll either be eating the flowers from the vase or devouring three rolls and butter before you've even ordered the meal. And there lurks danger.

Set yourself a time limit too, as the days of the three-hour lunch are over. You can always dream up a 3.30 appointment, complain your desk is piled up high, or that the MD is holding a management meeting later and you have to prepare. Always mention your excuse when making the date.

Do the same with a business dinner engagement – although it's sometimes more difficult. Plan your day's eating with the evening in mind; have an apple or something similar *before* the meal to stave off the pangs of potential roll-eating hunger; and save up your bonuses for that wine and after-dinner brandy if necessary. The menus starting on page 127 might help.

To quote a rather sexist story from my school days in relation to the *length* of lunches: when asked how long the assigned essay should be, our world-weary teacher replied: 'Like a woman's skirt – long enough to cover the subject, but short enough to make it interesting.' And so may it be with the business lunch or dinner.

SUITABLE RESTAURANTS AND CUISINES

And now for the possible choices if you're obliged to eat out at a restaurant. With only a few exceptions, most cuisines offer possibilities which will enable you to eat well without forcing you to fall off your dietary pedestal. (A handy tip: it's not customary to drink alcohol with many ethnic cuisines, so that could solve *one* problem.)

Grand and Costly

Haute cuisine and *nouvelle cuisine*, mainly French or international. Crudités to start are filling and unlimited (avoid dips), and there will always be something like grapefruit or melon. Any fish or seafood, meat or poultry, grilled preferably, and skinned if game or poultry. Avoid sauces. Limited potatoes, unlimited vegetables. Fresh fruit or fresh fruit salad (avoid alcohol- or syrup-based varieties) for afters.

Tony Aplin, Chairman of APA plc, comments on the problem of afters: he says 'Just coffee for me, please. It's amazing how everyone follows suit.' He believes that most business people realise they should be more weight-conscious, and the fact that somebody else has taken the lead eases their consciences. (Tony, incidentally, has shed 2 stone/12.6 kg, and has conscripted five of his senior executives on to the programme: the team has now lost over 10 stone/63 kg in all!)

Far Eastern

Chinese, Malaysian, Thai, Japanese. A fact not relevant to the diet, but worth considering: Charles Gray of Bache Prudential always checks his restaurants to see if they use MSG (monosodium glutamate). Many don't, and thus he avoids the dire consequences of 'Chinese Restaurant Syndrome', which can be unpleasant (too much MSG can have a temporary effect on the nervous system, and cause headaches). If eating Chinese, think in terms of Cantonese (the foods are steamed or boiled generally) rather than Peking, Shanghai or Szechuan (cuisines which use more oil and starch). A thin soup might be a good idea − a light broth or consommé with shreds of meat or vegetables cooked in it. Whole fish are steamed. Limit your rice input (boiled rather than fried), and enjoy the vast amounts of wok-cooked veg (a minimum of oil is used). Avoid all battered and deep-fried dishes. If eating Japanese, *sashimi* (raw fish) or certain *sushi* dishes (rice cooked with seaweed and topped with fish or veg etc) are naturals. Avoid noodle dishes − but any grilled fish or seafood is a wise choice. Non-syrupy fruit salad for afters, or fresh lychees or something similar.

Fish Restaurants

Anything goes here, except the batter-covered and fried choices.

Grilled or baked, from lobster to scampi, and brill to monkfish. Watch out for that tempting stack of bread and butter on the table, and avoid sauces. Drink your mineral water and hang on until the main dish arrives. There will be plenty of veg and salad. Avoid the dreaded chips, choosing boiled or baked potatoes. Fresh fruit or icecream for sweet — 2 oz (60 g) only of the latter.

Italian

Pasta is fine — wholewheat is best — but do watch the quantities. Cannelloni — large tubes of pasta stuffed with spinach and Ricotta cheese would be a good choice — but watch out for a heavy unctuous sauce. A large plate of *antipasti* or hors d'oeuvres — hot or cold salady bits and pieces — could be eaten as a main course. Parma ham — *prosciutto di Parma* — is often served with melon, figs or pears, and *bresaola* (dried salt beef) comes in very thin waxy slices. The Italian way with liver is superb — thin slices cooked with rosemary or sage (*grilled* for you) — and there are many veal dishes (again choose the plainest method of cooking). The famous *gelati* (icecream) or, perhaps better, *granite* (water ices, made without milk or cream), or fresh fruit for a sweet. Watch the quantities of everything, and keep away from those breadsticks and butter.

Greek

There are a number of salady starters, but stay away from those with cheese or beans — as well as the pâtés and pitta bread. Plain roast meat or charcoal-grilled kebabs would be a good choice, and there are some interesting vegetables. Fish are plain baked or grilled too. Avoid the sticky pastry puddings and, sadly, the Greek yoghurt (the best in the world), as it's made with full cream. Choose fresh fruit instead.

Indian

Tandoori dishes (chicken, mutton, lamb) are oven-cooked, and skinless — the perfect choice. Fish is occasionally available steamed or baked. Have some *raitha* to cool the taste-buds: it's natural yoghurt with chopped cucumber or mint and spices. There are a number of curd or cottage cheese dishes (*panir*) as well as interesting vegetables. Again, check on rice quantities and avoid those sickly sweets. Try fresh fruit (mangoes, often), ice-cream or a *lassi*, a salted yoghurt drink (there's a sugared version of the latter, but you don't want that).

Vegetarian

It isn't all nut cutlets and limp lettuce these days. But caution with the quantities − a lot of veggie restaurants feel that because they don't serve the dreaded *meat*, they can serve unlimited quantities of potatoes, corn, pasta, lentils and beans. Marvellous for the health-food industry, but murder for your waistline. Veg stews, salads (fruit *and* veg), and yoghurt are the best buys. And just because those chocolate cakes and brownies are offered in a vegetarian restaurant, they're no less dangerous than the sweet trolley at the Ritz.

West Indian

Here's an ethnic cuisine that's proving a welcome addition to the restaurant scene. Wonderful baked and grilled fish stuffed with onions and garlic. Try some of their more unusual vegetables: choco (a variety of squash or marrow, also called chayote), or akee (a fruit used as a veg, and wonderful with salt cod). Try a prawn dish with some brown rice, and choose mango, papaya or custard apples for afters.

Kosher

Latkes (potato pancakes), *kishka* or *helzel* (stuffed neck), and *kneidel* soup (with dumplings) may look irresistible, but danger lurks. Try the chopped liver − not too high a heap (cholesterol warning) − boiled or grilled chicken or chopped herring. And ask the waiter to remove that mile-high stack of rye bread; it's asking too much of you. There should be some appropriate salads, and have a fruit salad (make sure it's fresh) or sorbet for pud if you must.

Accompanying Liquids

As I have said, there's little emphasis on wines and spirits at Far Eastern, Indian, vegetarian or kosher restaurants, so you can get away with China tea at the Far Easterns group, *lassi* or water at the Indian, mineral water or lemon tea at the kosher and vegetarian restaurants.

Otherwise, have mineral waters, non-alcoholic wine or beer, spritzer, fruit juice or the wine of your choice. If fruit juice or wine, of course, *plan* for it, counting it as a serving in your weekly programme.

WHY NOT ENTERTAIN IN THE OFFICE?

A restaurant is only one of the possible choices available to you for business entertaining. Many firms now have canteens, dining rooms, or even just a part-time lady who whisks something together to order. Or, of course, you can order food *in*.

Alan Charvonia of Imperial Life entertains clients for lunch in his office. 'Smoked salmon with brown bread, lemon wedges plus champagne accomplishes miracles. No fussing with waiters and menus, no endless choices to be made. Clients really enjoy it, and you wouldn't believe how much more work is accomplished.'

Smoked salmon and champagne? Perfect for you if the quantities are correct and you've planned the day well. Don't go for sandwiches though, otherwise your bread and fat allotments will go haywire. Salad bars are widely seen nowadays, and you could order bowls of that to be brought in, served nicely and generously, with a little bread. Be careful with the dressings, though.

Perhaps you boast an executive dining room and a Cordon Bleu cook (more often than not she's tall, blonde and named

Fiona). Let her know your food programme and she'll take it from there. Trained cooks are acutely aware of weight-conscious clients, but are under-consulted. Her expertise and cooperation could be a tremendous help to you and your success.

MUST IT BE LUNCH OR DINNER?

I offer you a final thought about entertaining business clients while you're following a diet programme.

The world to me is made up of larks and owls. If you're a lark — rising early and unbearably cheerful at 6 am — you'll love the business breakfast. Owls, however, don't enter the world of the living until about 11 am, and to them an early mandatory breakfast is their idea of hell on earth (they'll be the lunch or dinner eaters!).

But for a lark, if you plan your daily programme with care, you can enjoy the legendary English breakfast, from juice and cereal, to eggs (not fried), kedgeree (not too much), kidneys and grilled kippers. All these goodies are part of your 'allowance', and can be eaten at any time of the day.

Lots of hotels and brasseries specialise now in breakfasts, especially in the City, and it's another meal at which you can get away with no booze.

BUSINESS BREAKFAST, LUNCH AND DINNER MENUS

To sum up on business entertaining:

1. Plan your meal as fully and as well in advance as possible.

2. Consult your partner.

3. Adjust your programme for that day to include the meal.

4. Stick to it.

BASIC PROGRAMME –
BUSINESS BREAKFAST DAY

Breakfast

4 oz (115 g) melon
1 oz (30 g) Cornflakes, with skimmed milk or yoghurt
1 scrambled egg, made with 1 level teaspoon low-fat
  spread and 1 oz (30 g) smoked salmon
1 oz (30 g) granary toast, with 1 level teaspoon low-fat
  spread
Tea or coffee unlimited – no sugar

Lunch

1 medium grapefruit
2 oz (60 g) tuna salad, with 1 level teaspoon mayonnaise
Coffee, lemon tea or mineral water

Dinner

Artichoke
3 oz (85 g) calf's liver, Italian-style
Runner beans, carrots, parsnips
8 oz (225 g) fresh fruit salad, with yoghurt if desired
Coffee, tea or mineral water

*How do I handle the all-too-frequent public appearances?
To reformed characters and streamlined physiques like
mine the question is ingenuous; you suffer in public as you
persevere in private, eschewing as opposed to chewing your
way through the menu. I do make a conscious point of
declining the bread and rolls whenever I eat out, just to
remind myself that I'm starting as I mean to carry on.*
Bryan Cowgill, Senior Television Executive

BONUS PROGRAMME – BUSINESS BREAKFAST DAY

Breakfast

4 oz (115 g) melon
2 oz (60 g) Bran Flakes, with skimmed milk or yoghurt
2-egg omelette, made with 1 level teaspoon low-fat
spread, plus 1 oz (30 g) grated cheese
1 oz (30 g) granary roll, with 1 level teaspoon fat-free
spread plus 1 level teaspoon no-sugar marmalade (see
page 43)
Coffee or lemon tea unlimited – no sugar

Bonuses: 1 extra carbohydrate + 1 extra protein

Lunch

2 oz (60 g) cold poached salmon, with 1 level teaspoon
mayonnaise
Runner beans, courgettes
5 oz (140 g) strawberries, with yoghurt if desired
Coffee, mineral water or diet drink

Dinner

1 medium grapefruit
3 oz (85 g) lean roast beef, with a little horseradish sauce
Peas, carrots, cauliflower
4 oz (115 g) fresh fruit salad
Coffee, tea or mineral water

BASIC PROGRAMME –
BUSINESS LUNCH DAY

Breakfast

4 fl. oz (115 ml) unsweetened orange juice
1 oz (30 g) Special K with skimmed milk or yoghurt, if
    desired.
Coffee or tea – no sugar

Lunch

4 oz (115 g) melon
4 oz (115 g) smoked salmon
1 oz (30 g) granary bread, with 1 level teaspoon low-fat
    spread
5 oz (140 g) strawberries, with yoghurt if desired
Coffee, tea or mineral water

Dinner

Artichoke
3 oz (85 g) roast veal
Green beans, carrots, cauliflower, with 2 level teaspoons
    low-fat spread
4 oz (115 g) fresh fruit salad
Coffee, lemon tea, mineral water

*'Don't read the list of starters – just ask for plain melon –
or whatever starter suits your purpose.'*
                              Tony Aplin, Chairman, APA

BONUS PROGRAMME –
BUSINESS LUNCH DAY

Breakfast

4 fl. oz (115 ml) unsweetened grapefruit juice
1 oz (30 g) unsweetened muesli, with skimmed milk or
   yoghurt
Coffee or tea unlimited – no sugar

Lunch

Asparagus
5 oz (140 g) lean roast beef, with a little horseradish
   sauce
6 oz (170 g) cooked potato
Carrots, beans, with 1 level teaspoon low-fat spread
5 oz (140 g) strawberries
3 fl. oz (85 g) claret
Coffee or mineral water

Bonuses: wine + 1 extra carbohydrate and 1 extra protein serving

Dinner

3 oz (85 g) Dover sole
Peas, courgettes
Mixed salad, with 2 level teaspoons vinaigrette
8 oz (225 g) fresh fruit salad
Coffee, mineral water or diet drink

BONUS PROGRAMME —
BUSINESS LUNCH DAY (ITALIAN)

Breakfast

1 pink grapefruit
1 oz (30 g) Rice Krispies, with skimmed milk or yoghurt
Coffee or tea unlimited — no sugar

Lunch

4 oz (115 g) Canteloupe melon
8 oz (225 g) lasagne, containing 4 oz (115 g) meat
   sauce (approximately) *or* a huge main-course dish of
   antipasti plus a breadstick(!)
Green salad, with 2 level teaspoons Italian dressing
6 fl. oz (170 ml) *vino*, red or white
Coffee or Pellegrino

**Bonuses: 2 × wine + 1 extra carbohydrate
possibly in the pasta. You're allowed less fat
today, because there will undoubtedly be
some in the lasagne.**

Dinner

4 oz (115 g) fresh fruit salad
3 oz (85 g) poached haddock
Peas, carrots, green beans
5 oz (140 g) raspberries, with yoghurt if desired
Coffee, lemon tea or mineral water

BONUS PROGRAMME – BUSINESS LUNCH DAY (KOSHER)

Breakfast

1 pink grapefruit
1 oz (30 g) granary toast, with as many grilled
    mushrooms and tomatoes as you want plus 1 level
    teaspoon fat-free spread
Coffee or tea unlimited – no sugar

Lunch

2 oz (60 g) chopped liver, with
1 oz (30 g) rye bread (you won't get dairy foods at a
    kosher restaurant)
5 oz (140 g) cooked chicken (no skin)
3 oz (85 g) boiled potato
Carrots, onions, peas, beans
8 oz (225 g) fresh fruit salad
Lemon tea, black coffee or mineral water

Bonuses: 1 carbohydrate and 1 protein serving

Dinner

Asparagus
3 oz (85 g) curd cheese
Mixed salad, with 2 level teaspoons of your favourite
    dressing
Peas and carrots
1 peach
Coffee, tea or mineral water

BASIC PROGRAMME –
BUSINESS DINNER DAY

Breakfast

1 grapefruit
1 oz (30 g) porridge made with skimmed milk (see page 36)
Coffee or tea unlimited – no sugar

Lunch

4 fl. oz (115 ml) unsweetened fruit juice
2-egg omelette, made with 1 level teaspoon low-fat spread
1 oz (30 g) granary roll, with 1 level teaspoon fat-free spread
Tea, coffee or diet drink

Dinner

4 oz (115 g) melon
5 oz (140 g) fillet steak
Cauliflower, peas, carrots, courgettes, with 1 level teaspoon low-fat spread
4 oz (115 g) fresh fruit salad
Coffee, tea or mineral water

'At parties, try to latch on to a good listener. You can't eat too much if you're talking all the time.'
David Quilter, Actor and Jogger

BONUS PROGRAMME – BUSINESS DINNER DAY

Breakfast

4 fl. oz (115 ml) unsweetened pineapple juice
1 poached egg on 1 oz (30 g) granary toast, with 1 level
teaspoon low-fat spread
Coffee or tea unlimited – no sugar

Lunch

3 oz (85 g) roast, skinless turkey
Brussels sprouts, parsnips, carrots
5 oz (140 g) strawberries
Coffee, tea or mineral water

Dinner

4 oz (115 g) melon
5 oz (140 g) lobster, with 2 level teaspoons dressing
3 oz (85 g) cooked potato
Peas, courgettes, green beans
2 oz (60 g) any flavour icecream, over
4 oz (115 g) fresh fruit salad
3 fl. oz (85 ml) wine
1½ fl. oz (45 ml) brandy
Coffee, tea or mineral water

Bonuses: wine, brandy, icecream + 2 extra protein servings (only 1 more bonus this week!)

BONUS PROGRAMME – BUSINESS DINNER DAY (INDIAN)

Breakfast

4 fl. oz (115 ml) unsweetened grapefruit juice
1 oz (30 g) unsweetened muesli, with 1 sliced medium peach, and skimmed milk
Coffee or tea unlimited – no sugar

Lunch

3 oz (85 g) Cheddar cheese salad
1 oz (30 g) granary roll, with 1 level teaspoon low-fat spread
5 oz (140 g) raspberries, in yoghurt if desired
Tea, coffee or diet drink

Dinner

Skip the *poppadoms* and *chapatis*
6 oz (170 g) chicken or lamb *tikka*
3 oz (85 g) saffron rice
Double order of *raitha*
Vegetables, as much as you like
1 pint (570 ml) lager or a *lassi* (see page 124)
4 oz (115 g) fresh fruit salad (make sure it's fresh: if it's got a gleaming maraschino cherry in the middle, it ain't) or a fresh mango

(You're only allowed 1 teaspoon low-fat spread today, as there's bound to be some used on the vegetables.)

Bonuses: 2 × lagers, 2 extra protein servings + 1 extra carbohydrate (and that's all your bonuses for the week used up!)

BONUS PROGRAMME –
BUSINESS DINNER DAY (CHINESE)

Breakfast

4 fl. oz (115 ml) unsweetened orange juice
1 oz (30 g) granary toast, with as many grilled tomatoes
and mushrooms as you like
Coffee or tea unlimited – no sugar

Lunch

4 oz (115 g) melon
3 oz (85 g) smoked salmon
1 oz (30 g) brown bread, with 1 level teaspoon fat-free
spread
4 oz (115 g) fresh fruit salad
Coffee or lemon tea

Dinner

Clear soup with meat and veg
6 oz (170 g) steamed or braised fish, or
Roast pork and duck, or 3 oz (85 g) of each
3 oz (85 g) plain boiled rice
Wok-cooked vegetables
4 oz (115 g) fresh fruit salad or fresh lychees, over 2 oz
(60 g) icecream
China tea or mineral water

(You're only allowed 1 teaspoon of fat today because the
vegetables will have been cooked in some.)

Bonuses: icecream + 2 extra protein
servings and 1 extra carbohydrate

BONUS PROGRAMME – BUSINESS RECEPTION

Breakfast

4 fl. oz (115 ml) unsweetened pineapple juice
1 oz (30 g) porridge made with skimmed milk (see page 36)
Coffee or tea unlimited – no sugar

Lunch

2-egg omelette made with 1 level teaspoon of low-fat spread
1 oz (30 g) granary roll with 1 level teaspoon of low-fat spread
Tea, coffee or diet drink

Evening Reception – Buffet

4 oz (115 g) melon
3 oz (85 g) roast beef
3 oz (85 g) roast chicken
3 oz (85 g) potato salad
As much salad and as many vegetables as you can pile on the plate
4 oz (115 g) fruit salad (no cream)
6 fl. oz (170 ml) red or white wine (augment white with Perrier)
Coffee or tea – no sugar

Bonuses: 2 × wine, 2 extra carbohydrates and 1 extra protein

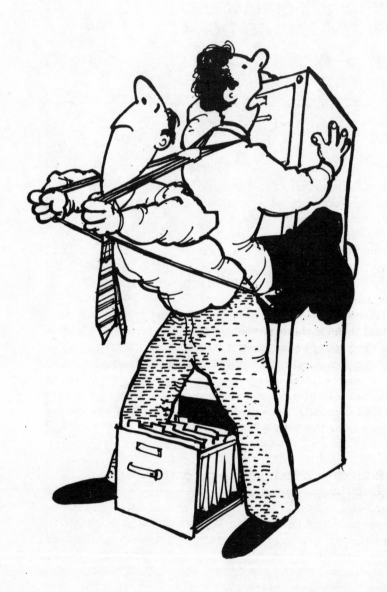

CHAPTER 7

Exercise – The Perfect Partner

The natural and perfect partner to an intelligent food programme is an intelligent exercise programme. And here again the watchword is moderation.

The scenario is classic. Middle-aged businessman seeing his doctor for a check-up. He's warned that he has to lose weight, give up smoking and start exercising. Otherwise, his future is uncertain and, in fact, limited. Panic stations. On to a starvation diet, a total ban on cigars and cigarettes, and a daily five-mile jog.

The starvation diet I've dealt with. Starving yourself will cause untold damage, both physiologically and emotionally, and is counter-productive in the long term – even in the mid term. Giving up smoking is a field in which I can claim no expertise at all. I can only confirm that clients of mine who have given up tobacco generally gain up to 10 per cent of their original weight within two months. Sometimes more. (A good food programme designed for the born-again non-smoker can be effective, but takes a good deal of application, especially in the initial stages.)

Suddenly setting off on a five-mile jog is an absolute disaster – literally. The average businessman, middle-aged and sedentary, generally confines his exercise to intermittent golf, occasional swimming, and even more occasional cricket, tennis and squash, or visits to the health club. The remainder of his sporting activities are confined to the spectator varieties (those on the sports pages rather than on the front or third pages of the tabloids). So donning a brand-new, fashionable tracksuit and jogging even a hundred yards will result in damage to the bones and under-used joints, tearing of muscles, dangerously high blood pressure, and, most seriously, a severe strain on the heart. Here again, as always, moderation is the keyword, and it's wise to check with your doctor before you begin any sort of exercise programme.

Caroline Cumberbatch runs a personal fitness service in Washington DC, which is a mirror image of my own service. I design a weight-control programme for clients based on their lifestyle and history, visit them regularly, and see that the programme is carried through successfully with plenty of personal back-up and advice. Caroline does exactly the same, but with fitness. She offers an exercise programme designed for her client, to be carried through regularly at home or office, with her or her colleague there to supervise. It's been a great success, with more business than they can handle – the majority of clients being male and middle aged (and financially sound).

She echoes my conviction that exercise is the natural partner to a weight-loss programme, and shared her experiences and comments:

'It is an undisputed fact that exercise aids enormously in the success of a slimming diet.

'By elevating the basic metabolic rate, calories are burned more efficiently, and that sluggish feeling goes. Secondly, the strengthening of the circulatory system (heart and lungs) through aerobic exercise leads to a lowering resting heart rate. Men overlook the fact that the heart is a muscle and, as such, needs to be exercised to keep its strength.

'Then we have the aesthetic improvement – a better shape through firmer muscles. You look better at any weight than a body defined by flab. And, most important, as weight is lost, some of it goes in the form of muscle. So exercise is essential in order to prevent exchanging a fat body for a soft thin one.

'In addition to the above life enhancers, you have more subtle benefits – more flexible joints, better posture, healthier skin tone and, last but not least, more confidence in your body.

'What exercise to do?

'Heavily overweight men need to get moving. Walking or swimming is best, or gentle aerobic exercise – sustained for not less than 30 minutes (1 hour is best) — around five times a week will work wonders. Results will be visible at three months, but you will feel better long before that.

'Men who have less to lose, up to 1 stone (6.3 kg), can try many different types of exercise — jogging, yoga, weight-training, aerobics. The important thing is to enjoy it. This may only come after some weeks, but what is essential is consistency and perseverance.

'The wonderful thing is that when the desired weight and fitness level is reached (ie when that five-mile walk is comfortable and pleasant), you can keep it with a minimum of three-weekly sessions, plus a good maintenance diet.

'I (naturally) recommend a personal trainer, if finances permit, just to help find the right exercise for the individual, and also so that correct stretching can be taught often, and added to, the aerobic work. (Muscles that have been contracted need to be stretched to keep them healthy and to relieve tension.) Otherwise, buy a good exercise book — a simple one with clear instructions. Buy one, if possible, written by a physiotherapist or physical therapist — and keep it simple.'

What I find fascinating is the emphasis on regularity — five times weekly initially, to three times weekly on maintenance; preferably 1 hour, but 30 minutes is acceptable. It rather backs up my own unprofessional theory that five minutes of daily waving my body about in pale imitation of the Royal Canadian Air Force exercises does me more good than a once-weekly jog, which I can't perform anyway (a result of my weak will and the flattest feet in the western hemisphere).

Personal fitness trainers are available in the UK and the States and elsewhere, and if you can afford it, they would be a good investment. Otherwise joining a health club or gym would be best. The initial cost of joining may be high, but the ultimate return can be well worth it.

The problem lies in the mid term. Your enthusiasm knows no bounds when you're shown over the premises: gleaming equipment, welcoming saunas, dedicated and muscled staff glowing with health and sun-bed tans. Yes, they will test you, and design an exercise programme just for you. Great. You join, and throw yourself into the programme with vim and vigour. After the first few weeks, you gradually find more pressing engagements that you can't postpone, or think that it's a bit chilly, or that you'd rather stay in bed just a bit longer. Your attendance lessens, and eventually you're too embarrassed to turn up at all. The answer is, as with everything in this book, perseverance. It'll pay off. A reputable health club or gym is a *great* aid for the attainment and maintenance of your fitness. The more frequent the attendance, the fitter the body (and, often, the lower the cost).

Otherwise, start your *own* programme. Take it gently at first, perhaps swimming regularly before or after work, or walking to work daily instead of taking a cab. If you use public transport, try getting off one or two stops earlier, and walking. Taking the stairs instead of the lift is another way of fitting some exercise into the working day. And try and fit in some of the exercises below as well.

I've always been somewhat cynical about the 'no pain, no gain' school of exercises. It strikes me that putting yourself through a pain barrier is senseless and smacks of the masochistic. I agree that exercise should be felt to be effective and that shambling along with your hands in your pockets to the local does not constitute exercise. But neither does getting a heart attack. An immoderate, over-energetic programme, whether in sport or exercise is no indication of either machismo or fitness. Unless you're a Daley Thompson clone, settle for a regular exercise programme that makes you feel good, raises your metabolic rate and increases your energy. You'll never lose weight by exercise alone (the loss of liquid through perspiration is immediately made up by the first drink you take), but combine exercise with an intelligent food programme and you're on to a real winner.

The following exercises, prepared for me by Karen Mottram, involve no pain (just perseverance), and will stretch you both mentally and physically. They're stretching, non-ballistic (non-bouncy) exercises which combine magnificently with your weight-loss programme. The stretching gets the muscles going gently, and because the exercises aren't bouncy, there is less danger of damage being done. As the weight drops off, the exercises done regularly will help re-align your whole body shape, keep you fit and energetic and out of the osteopath's waiting room.

STRETCHING EXERCISE ROUTINE

These exercises have been carefully and fully researched and are recognised as highly beneficial and completely safe for the average man. Firstly, though, a few words about the basics.

If you *bounce* while stretching, it confuses the muscles into contracting and relaxing violently, which causes tears and sometimes complete ruptures.

The exercises must be done with at least one bent leg — depending on the exercise. This prevents strain on the lower back, which is a highly vulnerable area. Keeping the knees bent when in a standing position takes the strain from the kneecaps — another vulnerable area.

All the stretches should be held for 15-20 seconds. Breathe *out* with the strain; breathe *in* as you relax. If any part of the body starts shaking with the strain, *stop immediately*. Stop if you feel any pain in the lower back. If the muscles relax, try and move a little further.

Start with a warm-up and then do all the exercises in the routine.

Warm Up

1. Stand, legs apart, knees bent, tummy in, bottom under, and shoulders down. This is the *basic starting position*. Stretch right arm above your head and rotate it backwards and then forwards in a clockwise circle. Do this eight times, then change arms and repeat.
2. In the starting position, lift and rotate the right shoulder forwards in a circular movement. Do this eight times, then reverse the direction of the circle eight times. Repeat with the other shoulder.
3. In the starting position, stretch your right arm up above your head. Bring it down to shoulder level out to the side, and repeat this movement eight times. Do the same with the left arm.
4. In the starting position, place your hands on your hips. Raise

the right hip eight times. Repeat with the left hip. NB. Keep your feet flat on the floor, and your upper body as still as possible. It's quite difficult!

5. In the starting position, with your hands on your hips, move your weight on to your left leg. Lift your right heel and, keeping the ball of the foot on the floor, rotate the right leg in a clockwise direction eight times. This is to get your ankle and knee moving. Repeat with left foot, eight times. Repeat exercise with both feet in an anti-clockwise direction.

6. March on the spot, keeping the upper body still, raising upper leg and knee to the horizontal position. NB. Make sure the heels return to the floor.

A. Side Stretch

In the starting position, rest right hand on side of right thigh. Straighten your left arm above your head, and lean towards your right side, taking support on your right hand. Feel the stretch on your left side. Repeat on the left side. NB Have your hips square and central, and *do not bounce*.

Progression. Sit cross-legged and place your right hand on the floor, about 4 inches (10 cm) from your right hip, with your elbow slightly bent. Lean over to the right, with your left hand stretched up and coming over your head. Do the same on the left. NB. Do not collapse the body. Always feel as though you are lifting from the head.

B. Hamstring Stretch (under thigh)

Lie on your back and push your tummy into the floor by pulling in the stomach muscles (to prevent your back arching). Bend your right leg, foot up to your bottom. Bring the left leg and knee into your body, clasping with both hands under the thigh (very important, as it takes any force off the knee). Slowly straighten the left leg until it is almost straight and bring towards head using arms clasped around under thigh. Do not *bounce*. Hold for 15-20 seconds, then repeat on right leg.

Progression. Sit on the floor with your legs slightly apart in front of you and bend your right leg. Reach over the straightened leg, lifting up through your stomach as you lean forward. Hold the stretch — *do not bounce*. Repeat with the other leg.

C. Groin Stretch (inner thigh)

Sit on the floor with your legs apart straight out in front of you, with your hands on the floor between your legs. Make sure your legs remain relaxed. Lean forward as far as you can, supporting yourself on your hands. You will only manage to move about 4 inches (10 cms) to start.

If it is really difficult, bring your legs closer together and bend your knees slightly. NB. Keep your knees pointing upwards.

Progression. Sit on the floor with the soles of your feet together and back straight as though you are a puppet, and gently push knees down towards the floor with your elbows. NB. Do not bounce, just go through the stretching process.

D. Quad Stretch (top of thigh)

Lie on the floor face down. Put left hand under chin, take right ankle with right hand, and pull into bottom. Feel the stretch. Keep knees together on the floor. Repeat on left leg.

Progression. Find a wall. Balance yourself against the wall with one hand, and do the same procedure with each leg alternately.

E. Calf Stretch

Stand with legs one in front of the other, hip distance apart. Bend the front knee and straighten the back leg, keeping your back heel on the floor and the body upright. Make sure the front knee is over your toes. Stretch, and repeat with the other leg. NB. Keep facing forward.

F. Final (Relaxing) Stretch

Kneel down and sit back on your heels. Reach up with your hands above your head, then reach forward and down so that your chest is lying on your thighs and your hands are on the floor (in the praying position). Make sure that your head and neck is relaxed. Hold the position for 5-8 seconds.

Finale

Stand up with legs together and arms by your side and do ten very easy star jumps — with your legs apart and arms out to the sides and then going back together again — making sure to bend your knees and land with heels flat on the floor.

HOW AND WHEN TO EXERCISE

This is strictly a question of personal preference and suitability — but it should never be after food. Morning people — the 'larks' — naturally choose the early morning, 'owls' prefer the evenings after work. There's no current overwhelming support for any one specific time. Some experts claim the mornings are more appropriate to increase the metabolism. Others disagree.

The controversy as to when is only matched by the 'how' argument. One fact which did strike me was the overnight affluence of osteopaths, chiropractors, bone specialists, and manipulators of every description. That this wave of prosperity occurred within weeks of the introduction of aerobics classes may be a coincidence, but I doubt it. The theory that the body must be tortured in order to benefit is somewhat masochistic in my opinion. It's certainly unnecessary. That's why I chose the above non-bouncy (non-ballistic) exercises. There's absolutely no pain involved, and no painfully expensive visits to your friendly neighbourhood bone specialist.

Whether in the morning or in the evening, aerobic or non-ballistic, at home or at the office, at the health club or gym, the vital ingredients yet again are planning, partner consultation and regularity. I cannot stress too strongly my conviction that a regular exercise regime, partnered by a sensible eating programme, is unbeatable. That slim, supple, toned-up body could be yours.

EXERCISING YOURSELF SLIM

The older you get, the longer you should exercise as you'll obviously not want to do anything too vigorous. The chart opposite will give you an idea of how many calories are used up during your regular 30-minute exercise sessions. I know The Businessman's Diet is based on weights and not calories, but as I said in Chapter 1, the Basic Programme is based on approximately 1,000 calories a day and the Bonus Programme contains around 1,500.

USING UP CALORIES

Activity (pursued with some enthusiasm)	Approx. Calories Used in 30 Minutes by a Man Weighing 11st 6 lb/ 160 lb/72.6 kg
Ballroom dancing	150
Cycling (slowly)	130
Golf	120
Rowing	400
Skiing	350
Squash	325
Tennis	260
Walking (slowly)	100
Walking (briskly)	170

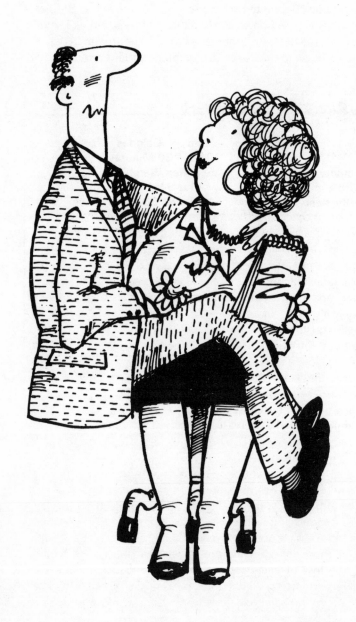

CHAPTER 8

'Harry, Darling, You Look Absolutely Marvellous!'

It's four to six weeks later — yet another early morning. Take a long look in the mirror. Nude, of course. After the loo and after a shower. Just like before you started on the diet.

It may not be Paul Newman staring imperiously back, and the bulging muscles of Sylvester Stallone are not to be seen, but it's not the same man of six weeks ago. It's you all right, but the new sleeker model with built-in energy and reserves of power — a leaner you that works and plays better, enjoys increased stamina, sleeps like a log, and exudes health and self-confidence.

Perhaps you've lost 10 or 15 pounds, or even more. Perhaps you're at your target — or well on the way. You've met the challenge and succeeded.

And it hasn't all been misery and deprivation. The skimmed milk isn't all that tasteless, you don't miss the peanuts and crisps that much, and the increased fruit and vegetables have gone down very well indeed. Even the drop in wine consumption has saved you money. In fact, you've got used to it. Well, I'm pleased that you have — for you'll be on it for the rest of your life.

It's no use trying to pretend that once you reached the weight you've aimed at, you can return to your previous eating and drinking habits. Reversion to your previous life will be a reversion to your previous weight. And along with the weight gain, all those tell-tale symptoms — the heartburn, the sleeplessness, the loss of energy, the exhaustion and irritability. And, most important, you'll lose the self-confidence and pride that your success has achieved. In the words of a well-known political leader — there is no alternative. Don't succumb to the 'Whoopee, school's out' syndrome — you'll wake up to regret it. Celebrate, by all means, but resolve you'll never return to your previous overweight lifestyle.

A PERSUASIVE FACTOR

A very welcome by-product of weight-loss and better health is the realisation that you're a great deal more visually attractive.

Because of your new body, you're buying new clothes that you previously wouldn't dare to wear. Because of the increase in your self-confidence, you exude an air of relaxed control that inspires admiration and even glances of sexual promise. No, I'm not going over the top. Your weight loss has changed a great many aspects of your life. Why I'm beating about the bush saying 'attractive' and 'visually pleasing', I really don't know. What I actually mean is that you're *sexier* — to others as well as yourself. You may not experience the doubtful joys of nubile young things throwing themselves at your feet, but you will enjoy more than the occasional admiring look from strangers and friends alike. Your family too will be delighted — and so they should be. You'll be with them for a lot longer, in better shape, and in a better mood.

I was fascinated to hear the view of Helena Amram of Helena International — the world's most exclusive (and expensive) marriage bureau — who knows more than most about sexual attraction and how slimness plays such an important part in relationships. She told me: 'One of the biggest turn-offs for most women is a man with a paunch.

'Most women, even independent ones, are looking for a man who can take care of them — not necessarily financially — but certainly emotionally. So who needs a man who can't take care of his own body? Of course, the same applies vice-versa. Confidence and a feeling of self-esteem is the ultimate attraction, and few men, or women, generate that if they feel they're carrying excess pounds. Besides, any man who's had too many expense-account lunches, or any woman who has spent her afternoons with her feet up on the sofa cradling the biscuit tin, is running considerable health risks.

'I wouldn't recommend anyone to look twice at a potential partner if they're more than a stone overweight − even if he has Henry Kissinger's brain, or she has Liz Taylor's eyes. Unless they're planning to do something about those unsexy lumps and bulges *fast*.'

This question of attractiveness is rarely mentioned out loud by men on a diet. The average man, certainly of my generation, would give his reasons for losing weight as better health, greater energy and stamina − even a smaller size in clothes. But he'd rather be stripped naked on the floor of the Stock Exchange than admit to a sexual motive.

That's where women have the advantage − they know themselves better and are able to express their true feelings without that false machismo pride that hampers the average man in so many of his personal relationships.

I can't count how many of my female clients have listed 'a new lover' or 'better sex' as reasons for losing weight, or 'My husband says he loves me the way I am, but I know he'd prefer me slimmer', or 'I want to be the centre of attention at parties, not sitting in the back as the jolly fat girl whom everyone likes'. Of course, everyone likes her − the other women especially. She presents no possible competition for their man's attention; not at that weight, for sure.

Behind the facade of the jolly fat person is a deeply unhappy and unfulfilled individual − the classic case of laughing on the outside, crying on the inside.

Let's all be more up front about the reasons for losing weight. What's wrong with men wanting to appear more sexy and attractive anyway? As a high-powered executive friend of mine notes: 'When you have lost 2½ stone after 20 years, the world marvels. It's worth four months' modest effort to get that adulation (at age 48) from men and girls of all ages − and it wasn't an effort after a few weeks.'

MAINTENANCE

It's never easy to change the eating habits of a lifetime. You're going to get a good amount of hassle from colleagues and a large amount of teasing from the family. You're still going to feel an appetite for the foods you're missing, and you're still going to enjoy the occasional treat that you shouldn't.

You won't turn into a dieting saint in four or six weeks, and thank the Lord for that. There's nothing quite as effective to stop conversation at a dinner table than boasting how well you've done on your diet. Let the weight loss speak for itself — it's quite apparent to everybody, even if they would sooner cut off their right arms than mention it.

If you've lost 10 - 14 lb (4.5 - 6.3 kg), but *haven't* reached your target weight, you're bang on course. The majority of men need to lose well over 21 lb (9.4 kg), and that will take longer than four weeks.

Try to aim for 1½ - 2½ lb (675 g - 1.1 kg) loss weekly, and pat yourself on the back if you're achieving that. Curb your inclination to relax your programme and reject the insidious feeling of giving up because 'Charlie told me I was looking a bit haggard'. If you're losing at the proper rate you're not looking haggard in the least. Perhaps Charlie himself is a bit flabby and there's more than a touch of envy in his remark. Keep your cool and keep on losing. It's yourself you have to please; it's yourself who has to succeed.

If you *have* reached your target weight in four weeks, congratulations. You've done remarkably well, and don't put yourself down by blushing coyly and muttering that you only had ten pounds to lose anyway. Losing that amount is as difficult to achieve for you as it is for another man to lose five stone. You're not competing with the chap opposite you on the tube, or your business rival, or your brother-in-law. You're putting the challenge to yourself; you're running against yourself in a sort of diet marathon. You're pleased that the man running with you crosses the finish line successfully. You're more than pleased that you've done it yourself. The weeks of training and planning have paid off. But just as a good runner can't relax, you can't relax either. The lessons you've taught yourself about yourself can never be forgotten or ignored. If you want to feel good about yourself, continue to look good, you're on it for life, but that life will be longer, fuller and much more enjoyable.

And if you *have* reached your target, now's the time to test yourself — new foods certainly, and new quantities possibly. You're still charting your food intake, you're still weighing where possible, and you're making certain you're having all the correct food in every category — no cutting down, no skipping and no cheating yourself.

Try an increased daily ration of bread for two weeks. No other changes, just the bread. If your weight holds steady, incorporate it into your programme. If the weight goes up, try another two weeks at half the extra quantity. Or try another ounce of protein for a couple of weeks, or more potato, or more pasta.

Never go below the minimum amount in any category, and you can't reduce one group of foods to have an increased portion of another. No cutting down on fruit, for instance, to increase the cereals. And certainly no increase in the amount of extras, for in that direction lies the dreaded chocolate bar syndrome, which means adding a *no-no* food into your programme, keeping your weight stable for a few weeks and then accepting that extra *no-no* as an integral ingredient to your programme. Crime does *not* pay, and the weight will come back on — it may be in two weeks or four, but it will return! You can test yourself in every food category *except* the *no-nos* and bonuses. Plan your test and chart the results.

If you haven't succeeded on the programme, or you've had to give up for any reason, don't feel guilty. There's always tomorrow — but don't wait until then. Take a positive step and start again today. The investment in time and planning is minimal — the rewards are great.

And now a brief re-cap of the main points to remember.

1. Eat everything you should from every category.

2. Never *under*-eat.

3. Don't hold foods over from one day to another.

4. Eat when it suits you, but you must eat everything required in a 24-hour period.

5. Consult your partner about every aspect of your food programme – in unity there is strength!

6. Weigh everything if and when you can. Don't guess – you'll always under-estimate.

7. Chart everything – how much, when and what.

8. Weigh yourself once weekly – same scale, same time, same place.

9. If you over-do it, forget the guilt and start again the next day.

10. Enjoy the extras, but don't exceed the maximum allowed.

11. Treat your diet seriously – it's not a giggle, but, alternatively, don't get obsessive.

Congratulations on meeting the challenge, and best wishes for your continued success.

The Diet Centre

All of us at Brook Green Diet Centre believe that weight loss and maintenance of that weight loss is a major lifestyle alteration. It cannot be approached by guarantees of overnight losses or miraculous cures. We provide no pills, no injections, no supplements, no sensational discoveries and we are not financed by any outside commercial organisations. In short, we offer no Miracle Cures.

What we do provide is a programme of close medical supervision, behaviour modification and nutritional counselling. Programmes are individually tailored to the client's lifestyle (after a comprehensive initial consultation) and no two programmes are alike. Regular counselling plays a vital role both during the Programme and after the target weight is achieved. Our clients, both personal and corporate, enjoy total confidentiality.

The Designer Weight Control Division provides an alternative service — we bring the Programme to you. Whether at your home or office, it's discreet, time-saving and very popular with our clients. This service is suitable for individuals and small groups.

If you want to lose weight and maintain that weight loss with an intelligent programme that's medically-supervised, individually tailored and effective, please get in touch. We'd be delighted to hear from you and have a chat.

THE DIET CENTRE

Designer Weight Control

56 Brook Green, London, W6
Telephone: 01-602 8184

Directors:
Dr. Sally Birkett, Michael Teff, Margaret Birkett

Index

(P) signifies food items prohibited in the Basic Diet;
(A) signifies food items allowed in the Basic and/or Bonus Diets.